Basic Guide to Dental Materials

T0260710

To my dear husband Padraig and sweet daughter Abigail, without whose love and attention I would have finished this book in half the time.

BASIC GUIDE TO DENTAL MATERIALS

Carmen Scheller-Sheridan

C.D.A., R.D.N., Dip. Ad. Ed., M.A.

Dental Nurse Tutor
Dublin Dental School and Hospital
Trinity College Dublin
Republic of Ireland

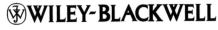
A John Wiley & Sons, Ltd., Publication

This edition first published 2010
© 2010 Carmen Scheller-Sheridan

Blackwell Publishing was acquired by John Wiley & Sons in February 2007.
Blackwell's publishing programme has been merged with Wiley's global Scientific, Technical,
and Medical business to form Wiley-Blackwell.

Registered office
John Wiley & Sons Ltd, The Atrium, Southern Gate, Chichester, West Sussex, PO19 8SQ,
United Kingdom

Editorial offices
9600 Garsington Road, Oxford, OX4 2DQ, United Kingdom
2121 State Avenue, Ames, Iowa 50014-8300, USA

For details of our global editorial offices, for customer services and for information about how to
apply for permission to reuse the copyright material in this book please see our website at
www.wiley.com/wiley-blackwell.

The right of the author to be identified as the author of this work has been asserted in accordance
with the Copyright, Designs and Patents Act 1988.

Library of Congress Cataloging-in-Publication Data

Scheller-Sheridan, Carmen.
Basic guide to dental materials / Carmen Scheller-Sheridan.
p. ; cm.
Includes bibliographical references and index.
ISBN 978-1-4051-6746-8 (pbk. : alk. paper)   1. Dental materials.   I. Title.
[DNLM: 1. Dental Materials. WU 190 S322b 2010]
RK652.5.S34 2010
617.6'95–dc22
2009037333

A catalogue record for this book is available from the British Library.

Set in 10/12.5 pt Sabon by Aptara® Inc., New Delhi, India
Printed in Singapore

1   2010

Contents

Preface: How to use this book

This guide is a supplemental resource to use alongside practical training and experiences. It works well in conjunction with *Basic Guide to Dental Instruments* (Scheller, 2006), which is also available in the Basic Guide series. Many instruments are referred to but not pictured, as the focus of this text is dental materials.

Basic Guide to Dental Materials has been written for anyone working or studying within the dental profession, particularly aimed at dental care professionals. It may be used as a study aid or within the dental surgery as a reference guide. It is not meant to be a comprehensive resource and needs to be used alongside study notes and other more comprehensive texts where appropriate.

Dental materials have been categorised by their usage in this text, and as many materials have multiple uses they are featured in multiple chapters. The first two chapters contain essential background information on dental materials, and all other chapters should be read as required in relevant circumstances. Each chapter follows the same format, with definitions, material properties, advantages, disadvantages, trade names, manipulation instructions, manipulation photos and mixing, working and setting times. It is important that the reader understands that although every effort was made to produce manipulation instructions and mixing, working and setting times, these properties may vary between manufacturers. It is the responsibility of the dental professional to consult manufacturer's instructions to ensure a comprehensive understanding of specific material properties.

This book is a UK publication where intraoral duties including the placement of dental materials have not yet been introduced as a skill of the dental nurse/dental assistant at the time of publication. In the event that these duties are introduced or in those areas of the world where they are practised, the individual must consult other references for information in relation to the clinical placement of dental materials.

Dental instrument and materials set-ups are included in each chapter. They only encompass what is required for the manipulation of the dental material and are not meant to be comprehensive for each procedure. Comprehensive procedure set-ups may be found in *Basic Guide to Dental Instruments* (Scheller, 2006).

Dental materials are ever changing. Continued professional development is essential to maintaining the most current knowledge of available products.

It is the responsibility of each member of the dental team to continuously review and update the knowledge required to work with the dental materials in the surgery. **It is imperative to follow the manufacturer's instructions when working with any dental material.** It would be impossible to create a text with every material by every manufacturer, so one material has been highlighted for manipulation and photography purposes. The author does not endorse using any specific dental material.

It is essential that good health and safety, and infection control standards are practiced when working with dental materials. Where possible, these have been mentioned throughout the text. If you have any queries in relation to these areas consult your surgery policies or legislative bodies for appropriate regulations and legislation in your area.

REFERENCE

Scheller, C. (2006) *Basic Guide to Dental Instruments*. Oxford: Blackwell Publishing Ltd.

Acknowledgements

I would like to thank the many people who helped with the editing and development of this guide to dental materials including: Professor Robert Ireland, Ms. Tina Gorman, Dr. Frank Quinn, Dr. Osama Omer, Dr. Owen Fleetwood, Ms. Joan Brennan, Mr. Declan Byrne, Dr. Richard Pilkington, Ms. Helen Phipps and Ms. Catherine Waldron. Thanks to Mr. Mark Thompson for taking many of the pictures within this text and to the following for helping to gather materials and allowing me to photograph them: Louise Boyd, Madonna Bell, Daniel Doyle and Rebecca Hayden.

I would also like to thank the following companies who supplied photographs and/or dental materials for photography purposes:

3M ESPE
Bosworth
Heraeus Dental
Kerr
Keystone
Premier Dental Products Company
Promed
Pulpdent Corporation
SDI
Waterpik
Whipmix

Chapter 1
Introduction

THE DENTAL TEAM

Dental materials are used daily in the dental surgery. It is imperative that the dental team is knowledgeable in relation to a variety of dental materials and their distinguishing characteristics. Biocompatibility, durability, aesthetics and cost must all be taken into account when choosing a dental material. New dental materials are introduced to the market continually, and it is the responsibility of the dental team to keep their knowledge base up to date through Continual Professional Development (CPD) opportunities.

Loss of, or damage to tooth structure requires the use of a variety of dental materials to repair and/or replace the missing structure. Missing tooth structure may be as a result of trauma, caries (decay) or various other causes. Dental materials are often categorised by their usage, as they will be in this text.

THE DENTAL NURSE

The role of the dental nurse in relation to dental materials is important. The dental nurse must be knowledgeable in the areas of instrument set-up, armamentarium (complete set-up for treatment), mixing, manipulation, proper disposal of used instruments and materials, material constituents, material storage, stock maintenance and health and safety in relation to the materials.

In areas of the world where dental nurses or dental assistants have intraoral responsibilities including the placement of dental materials, their knowledge must be expanded to include the comprehensive understanding of material placement, which is not included in this text.

DENTAL MATERIALS – DISPENSING, MANIPULATION AND APPLICATION

Dispensing

Dental materials are dispensed in various forms as shown below:

A. Two-paste systems (Figure 1.1a and 1.1b)

B. Powder and liquid form (Figure 1.2)

C. Capsule form (Figure 1.3)

D. Compule form (Figure 1.4)

E. Syringe form (Figure 1.5)

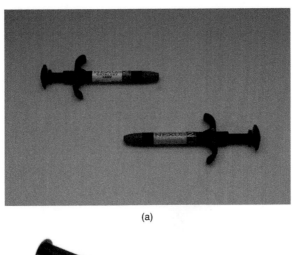

(a)

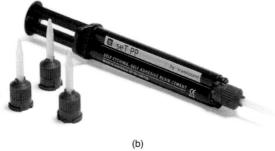

(b)

Figure 1.1 Two-paste system.

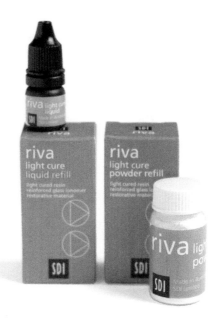

Figure 1.2 Powder and liquid form.

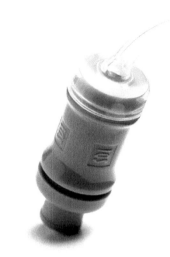

Figure 1.3 Capsule form.

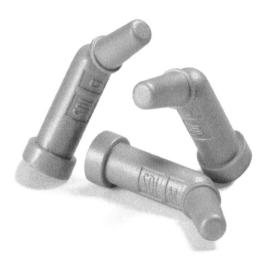

Figure 1.4 Compule form.

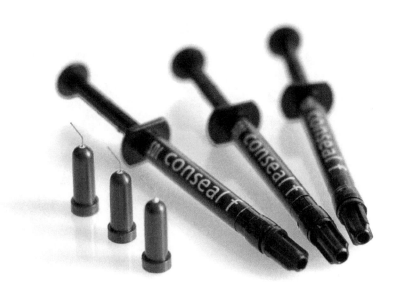

Figure 1.5 Syringe form.

Both two-paste systems and powder and liquid forms are manually manipulated, whilst the capsule form is preloaded with the exact ratios of materials and is mechanically manipulated. The compule and syringe forms are preloaded and ready to be dispensed with no mixing required (trituration may be required).

Mixing

Manual manipulation requires using a mixing spatula and some type of mixing surface.

Various mixing spatulas, which will be referred to within this text, are depicted in Figure 1.6.

A. Wooden-handled spatula

B. Weston spatula

C. Broad-bladed spatula

D. Plastic spatula

E. Fishtail spatula

F. Plaster spatula

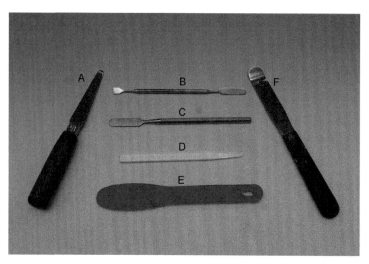

Figure 1.6 Mixing spatulas.

Mixing surfaces

Figure 1.7 depicts various mixing surfaces, which will be referred to within this text.

A. Dispensing well (can be used in conjunction with an amber shield that slides over the wells to shield light-sensitive materials from the light)

B. Glass dappen dish

C. Waxed paper pad (available in various sizes)

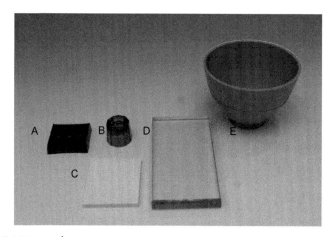

Figure 1.7 Mixing surfaces.

D. Glass slab

E. Flexible mixing bowl

Applicators

Figure 1.8 depicts various applicators, which will be referred to within this text.

A. Disposable brush

B. Disposable applicator

C. Calcium hydroxide applicator

D. Teflon-tipped flat plastic

E. Flat plastic

F. Amalgam carrier

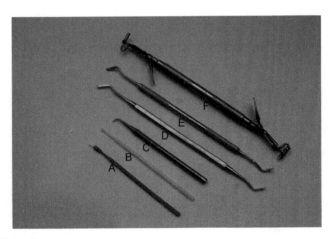

Figure 1.8 Applicators.

DISPENSING POWDER AND LIQUID

The powder and liquid forms of dental materials require the dental nurse to take care when dispensing, ensuring the correct amount of material is dispensed following the manufacturer's instructions.

Altering the ratios of dispensed materials will adversely affect the final mix, properties and behaviour of the dental material.

When dispensing powder that is supplied with a powder scoop

- Always fluff the powder prior to dispensing by shaking the bottle with the lid intact
- Dispense using the supplied powder scoop following the manufacturers instructions
- If the bottle has a ledge, use this to level the powder in the scoop. (Figures 1.9a–1.9d)
- If the bottle does not have a ledge, use a sterile spatula to level the powder in the scoop. (Figures 1.10a–1.10d)
- Replace the cap on the bottle immediately

When dispensing liquid

- Do not dispense until ready to use
- Hold the bottle perpendicular to the mixing surface (Figure 1.11)

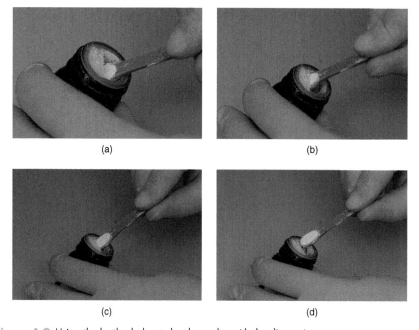

(a)   (b)

(c)   (d)

Figure 1.9 Using the bottles ledge to level powder with the dispensing scoop.

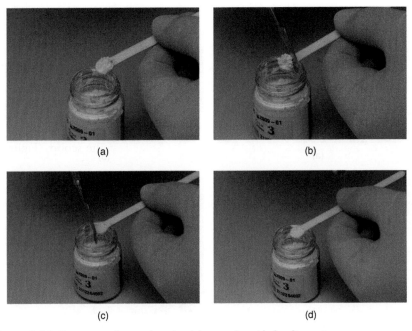

(a)

(b)

(c)

(d)

Figure 1.10 Using a sterile spatula to level the powder with the dispensing scoop.

- Depending on the dispensing system, the dental nurse will gently squeeze the bottle until one drop is released, then release the pressure and repeat the process until the desired amount of drops are dispensed. For calibrated dispensing systems, hold the bottle vertically until a drop is released from the bottle (Figures 1.12a–1.12d)
- Replace the cap on the bottle immediately

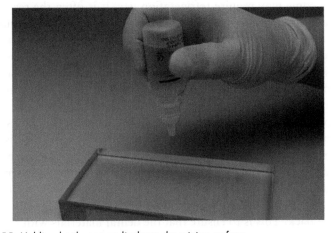

Figure 1.11 Holding bottle perpendicular to the mixing surface.

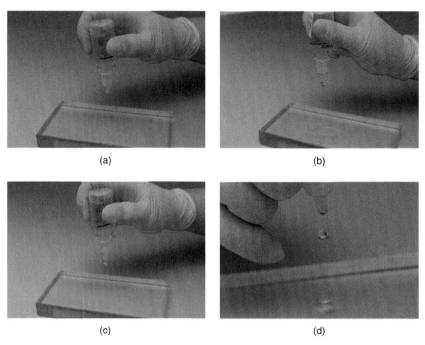

(a)   (b)

(c)   (d)

Figure 1.12 Dispensing liquid.

INVENTORY AND STORAGE OF DENTAL MATERIALS

It is important that the dental nurse takes care when ordering and storing dental materials. Dental materials must be stored as per the manufacturer's instructions, some may require refrigeration, etc. It is often the responsibility of the dental nurse to maintain the stock within a surgery. Dental nurses must familiarise themselves with the amounts of specific materials consumed and keep an adequate supply. 'Overstocking' should be avoided as it costs money and increases waste. Dental materials have an expiry date, and if they are not used within this time, they must be discarded. There should be a list kept of items that need reordering, and it is imperative to restock a supply when it is close to depletion. Running short or out of dental materials is unnecessary with proper planning, management and stock control. When new stock is received into the dental surgery, it is often the responsibility of the dental nurse to ensure that the order is complete, to check that the amount charged is correct and to put the stock in its place. When putting away dental materials, ensure that the stock is rotated and that the dental materials with the longest expiry date are placed to the back. This is to ensure that the dental materials with the shortest expiry date are used first.

TYPES OF RESTORATIONS

Before discussing the various types and properties of individual dental materials, it is useful to discuss the various types of restorations that will be referred to within this text in relation to dental materials.

A **direct restoration** is a restoration prepared for immediate placement in the mouth of the patient and does not require any external fabrication; they are frequently referred to as 'fillings'. Direct restorations require a sufficient amount of tooth surface to support the filling material and can be undertaken quickly and relatively inexpensively. Amalgam or resin composites are the materials most often used for direct restorations.

An **indirect restoration** is one that is processed and fabricated outside of the oral cavity, most often in a dental laboratory. This type of restoration requires an adhesive and/or a type of thin dental cement (luting material) to allow it to be retained in or adhere (stick) to the prepared tooth structure; examples are gold or porcelain inlays or onlays.

A **fixed restoration** or **fixed appliance** is one that is intended to remain in the mouth and is not routinely removed by the patient. It may be for an indefinite period of time, such as a crown or a bridge, or for a defined period of time, such as a space maintainer or a fixed orthodontic appliance.

A **removable appliance or prosthesis** is a dental appliance that is used to perform a specific function; for example, to replace teeth – a full denture, or a Hawley orthodontic appliance, which is used to prevent the movement of teeth and can be removed on a routine basis by the patient for cleaning or by the dentist or orthodontist for adjustment.

An **inlay** is an indirect restoration that is made to fit into a prepared cavity. It restores one or more surfaces of a tooth and may possibly include one or more cusps: it is usually made of gold, porcelain, or resin composite.

An **onlay** is an indirect restoration that replaces one or more cusps and adjoining occlusal surfaces of a tooth: it is usually made of gold, porcelain, or resin composite.

A **crown** is an indirect restoration that may be referred to by some patients as a 'cap'. It can cover the entire tooth or part of the coronal portion of the tooth. A crown is often indicated when the shape, function, or appearance of a tooth needs to be improved. Crowns that are not visible at the back of the mouth are often made of metal to provide adequate strength; those at the front of the mouth are usually made of porcelain or metal with porcelain bonded to the outer (visible) surface for aesthetic reasons.

A **bridge** or **'fixed partial denture'** is an indirect restoration that functions to replace one or more missing teeth. It is cemented to one or more adjacent teeth. The portion of the bridge that replaces some or the entire coronal portion of the supporting natural tooth is termed the *retainer*; the tooth to which the retainer is cemented is called the *abutment tooth*, and the part of the bridge that replaces the missing tooth is termed the *pontic*. Each pontic and retainer is termed a *unit*. It is the combination of the pontics and abutments that constitutes a bridge. Bridges can be fabricated from a variety of dental materials, and there are many different designs.

A **veneer** is a restoration that most commonly replaces the facial aspect of anterior teeth to improve the aesthetic appearance. Veneers may be fabricated indirectly in the laboratory and these are most often made of porcelain, or they can be fabricated directly in the mouth and these are made of resin composite.

A **denture** is a removable, indirect appliance whose function is to replace one or more teeth. Dentures may be classified as partial or complete. A **partial denture** replaces one or more teeth, and is retained in position by contact with the patient's natural teeth and supporting tissues. The frame of a partial denture may be made from acrylic, metals (chromium, cobalt and nickel) or a combination of both. Clasps may provide additional retention and can be used to anchor the partial denture to the patient's natural teeth. A **complete** or **full denture** is indicated when the patient has no teeth (edentulous) in one or both arches. The action of the patient's muscles and the surrounding tissue structure maintain the complete denture in place. An **overdenture** is a denture, usually a complete denture, that is fabricated to rest over dental implants or retained roots of natural teeth.

A **dental implant** is a replacement for the root of a natural tooth. It is placed within the jawbone. Dental implants can be fabricated from a variety of materials, such as titanium and titanium alloy. An implant is used to support a crown, bridge or denture to replace one or more missing teeth.

As summarised above, there are many different types of restorations and appliances that are indicated to restore the masticatory function and appearance of the patient. Each situation will dictate the need for a specific dental material to be used. It is the responsibility and duty of all members of the dental team to understand the implications, properties and appropriate manipulation of these dental materials in order to deliver the best oral health care to the patient.

Chapter 2
Dental materials' properties

The properties of dental materials are important to the dental professional when deciding how they are indicated in use. When selecting a dental material, there are many influences that must be taken into account. These include:

- the patient's medical history
- appearance
- cost
- the oral cavity environment
- the degree of masticatory force
- contact effects on oral tissues
- toxic effects in the event of ingestion and inhalation

This chapter aims to define some of the important terms used in relation to the properties of dental materials that must be taken into consideration during their selection. This is not meant to be an exhaustive list of terms; there are many good dental dictionaries available for reference. If you need further information, see the *Further reading* section at the end of this chapter.

ACIDITY

Dental materials can react to different acidities in the oral cavity. The pH of the oral cavity is normally around 7.0 (7.5 is neutral). Extrinsic sources (e.g. foods) may change the acidic properties. Saliva acts as a natural buffer and aids in reducing the acidity of the oral cavity. It is important for dental professionals to understand how different levels of acidity affect dental materials, as this determines the use and usability (the ease of use) of the dental material. The acidity of dental materials can also affect the oral cavity and surrounding tissues, which is also important for the dental team to understand.

ADHESION

Adhesion can be chemical or physical and relates to the way two unlike substances are held together.

AESTHETICS

Aesthetics refers to the pleasant appearance of the dental material once placed in the patient's oral cavity. Some materials, such as composite, allow the operator to choose the shade or colour of the material used in order to closely match it to the natural colour of the tooth.

BIOCOMPATIBILITY

Biocompatibility is the biologic response of the body to the use of a specific material. Responses may include irritation, sensitivity and toxicity. A biocompatible material will not cause a negative response, such as sensitivity, irritation or toxicity to the human body.

BITING FORCE

Dental materials must have adequate mechanical properties (strength) to resist temporary change due to masicatory forces and not be permanently deformed.

CORROSION

Corrosion occurs when two dissimilar materials are in contact or are surrounded by a conductive fluid, e.g. saliva, which results in degradation of the metal from a chemical reaction.

CREEP

Creep refers to the distortion that occurs in a material (e.g. metal) over a period of time when subjected to a continuous load (e.g. amalgam causing a cuspal fracture).

DIMENSIONAL CHANGE

Dimensional change refers to the shrinkage or expansion of dental materials on setting in response to stimuli such as heat, light curing and cold. Accuracy

DENTAL MATERIALS' PROPERTIES

of dental restorations is dependent on the dimensional change of the dental materials used directly or in conjunction during its fabrication (e.g. impression materials during the fabrication of a crown). Chemical reactions and temperature changes are two common factors that may result in the dimensional change of a material.

ELASTICITY

Elasticity refers to the property of a dental material which allows its dimensions to change when a force is applied and its ability to return to normal state once the force is removed.

FLOW

Flow refers to the viscosity of the dental material or the deformation of the material when undergoing force (creep), which is insufficient to break the material.

GALVANISM

Galvanism is the sensation that a patient can feel as a result of two dissimilar metals within their mouth. An example of this can be the sensation that a patient feels when a piece of tin foil comes in contact with a metal crown.

HARDNESS

Hardness of a dental material refers to its resistance to dimensional changes, scratches or indentations.

MICROLEAKAGE

Microleakage refers to the entrance of fluids (e.g. saliva) into the microscopic space existing between the tooth tissue and the dental material. When a tooth is prepared for a restoration, dentine may be exposed. Dentine is composed of tubules, which allows fluid to make its way in between the restoration and tooth surface. This fluid may travel down the dentinal tubules, which may result in damage to the pulp, decay surrounding the restoration, discolouration or insensitivity.

Microleakage may be reduced or temporarily avoided by the use of cavity varnish. Varnish may be applied to the cavity preparation, sealing the tubules. Varnish has been largely replaced by the use of bonding agents. Chemical or mechanical means of bonding are also used to reduce the risk of microleakage.

RETENTION

Retention of dental materials can be mechanical, chemical or a combination of both. Retention refers to the way in which a dental material adheres to the tooth structure. **Mechanical retention** of dental materials is achieved by the operator preparing the preparation of the tooth in such a way that the material is locked into place or making the tooth microscopically rough. **Chemical retention** is the result of a chemical reaction between the tooth structure and the dental material in order for it to adhere.

SOLUBILITY

Solubility refers to how a material dissolves when present in certain environments.

THERMAL CONDUCTIVITY

Dental materials have varying levels of their ability to conduct heat. Metals have a higher thermal conductivity than resins or porcelain. Hence, a patient with an amalgam restoration may be temporarily sensitive to heat changes within the oral cavity.

TRANSLUCENCY

Translucency is a natural attribute of a tooth and is desirable to achieve during the restoration of teeth. It refers to the amount of light that can penetrate the surface of the tooth. It is natural for the incisal edges of anterior teeth to appear more translucent than the cervical area as it is thinner.

VISCOSITY

Viscosity refers to the flowability of a dental material.

WETTABILITY

Wettability refers to the flow of a dental material over a solid surface.

FURTHER READING

Ireland, R. (Forthcoming) *Oxford Dictionary of Dentistry*. Oxford: Oxford University Press.

Chapter 3
Temporary restorative materials

Certain dental cements mixed to a base or putty-like consistency can be used as **temporary restorative materials,** and there are other materials available that have temporary filling as their main function.

Provisional or temporary crown materials are also considered temporary restorative materials but will not be discussed in this chapter.

CAVIT™

CAVIT™ (3M ESPE) is a self-cure, temporary restorative material (Figure 3.1).

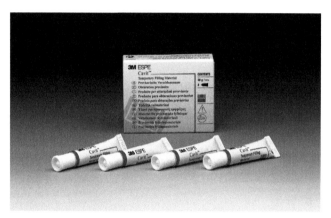

Figure 3.1 CAVIT™ – 3M ESPE.

Material constituents/composition

- Zinc oxide
- Calcium sulphate
- Barium sulphate
- Talc
- Ethylene bis(oxyethylene) diacetate
- Zinc sulphate
- Poly(vinyl acetate)

TEMPORARY RESTORATIVE MATERIALS

Properties

- Self-cure
- Packable
- Radiopaque
- Available in light curable form

Advantages

- No manipulation required
- Easy to place

Disadvantages

- Is not suitable for 'shallow' restorations

Indications and contraindications for use

Indications
- Temporary restorations
- Inlay and onlay temporary restorations

Contraindications
- Not indicated for use in areas less than 3–5 millimetres thick

Manipulation

Wearing personal protective equipment.
  Once the tooth is prepared for restoration:

  Step 1

  - Dispense the required amount of CAVIT™ on a waxed paper pad using a sterile instrument

Step 2

- Transfer to the operator with a flat plastic instrument or operators instrument of choice

Step 3

- The operator will place the material into the cavity preparation
- Be prepared with a piece of gauze to wipe excess material from the blunt instrument

Step 4

- Dispose of any waste material and waxed paper pad in the contaminated waste bin (Figure 3.2)

Mixing time

- No mixing required

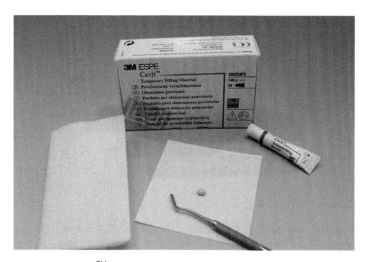

Figure 3.2 Step 1 – CAVIT™ – 3M ESPE dispensed.

Instruments and materials used in set-up

Materials used in set-up:

- Waxed paper pad
- CAVIT™ material
- Flat plastic instrument

ZINC OXIDE EUGENOL

Zinc oxide eugenol (ZOE) may be used as a base, a temporary restorative material, a temporary luting agent, impression material, bite registration material, an endodontic sealer or a periodontal dressing. In this chapter, ZOE will be discussed in the context of a *temporary filling material*. ZOE cements are oil-based cements that have a sedative effect on the pulp.

Material constituents/composition

Available in powder and liquid form, two-paste system and capsule form.

Powder (base)	Liquid (acid)
Zinc oxide	Eugenol
White resin	Water
Zinc stearate	Oils
Zinc acetate	

ZOE type cements are also available in a non-eugenol form (does not contain eugenol), which is suitable for use with patients having a sensitivity to eugenol. It is also suitable for use with resin adhesive restorations. The non-eugenol form contains oils rather than eugenol.

ZOE is available in two forms. **Type II** is reinforced and contains methyl methacrylate or alumina in the powder form and eugenol and ortho-ethoxy benzoic acid in the liquid form. These additions reduce the solubility and improve the strength of the material. **Type I** contains none of these additional materials, thereby reducing the strength and making it more suitable for temporary restorations.

TEMPORARY RESTORATIVE MATERIALS

Properties

- Type I and Type II are available
- Type I low strength, Type II (reinforced) moderate strength
- Neutral properties
- Moisture is required for setting

Advantages

- Antimicrobial – soothing effect on the pulp
- Good sealing ability

Disadvantages

- Type I has a high solubility and Type II has a moderate to low solubility
- Does not release fluoride
- Type I has a lower strength than Type II, which has moderate strength
- Does not adhere well to enamel or dentine

Indications and contraindications for use

Indications
- Base
- Temporary filling material
- Luting cement
- Periodontal dressing
- Temporary cement
- Bite registration material

Contraindications
- Not to be used in conjunction with resin composites, as the eugenol contained in zinc oxide eugenol retards the setting

Trade names

Trade name	Manufacturer
B&T®	Dentsply/Caulk
IRM®	Dentsply/Caulk
Kalzinol	Dentsply/Caulk
Reinforced ZOE Cement (Figure 3.3a)	Master-Dent
Sedanol	Dentsply/Caulk

Manipulation (Figures 3.3b–d)

Wearing personal protective equipment.
  Powder/liquid:

Step 1

- The operator will prepare and isolate the tooth appropriately

Step 2

- Dispense the material immediately prior to use

Step 3

- Powder to liquid ratio of 3:1
- Fluff powder bottle with cap in place (this provides a more consistent volume of powder in each scoop)
- Dispense powder onto waxed paper pad (using the measuring scoop, if provided)
- Replace the lid on the powder bottle immediately after dispensing

Step 4

- Divide the zinc oxide eugenol powder into four equal portions using the broad-bladed spatula (Figure 3.3b)

Step 5

- Dispense liquid, holding it perpendicular to the waxed paper pad; dispense as per the manufacturer's instructions. A ratio of approximately

3:1 powder to liquid should be used (follow the manufacturer's instructions as this may vary)

- Replace the dropper to the bottle

Step 6

- Incorporate one powder measure into the dispensed liquid. Use the broad part of the spatula to mix in the powder using a 'stropping motion'. The mix may initially appear thick or crumbly; keep mixing with a stropping motion as this will bring out the oil in the mixture, bringing the mix to the desired consistency

Step 7

- Repeat step 6 until the desired consistency is met, which is a putty-like mixture that can be rolled into the shape of a rope or a ball using the spatula (Figure 3.3d)

Step 8

- Pass the zinc oxide eugenol material to the operator on the waxed paper pad with the operator's choice of hand instrument (usually flat plastic instrument or condenser/plugger)
- Leave a small amount of powder for the operator, as it may be used as a separator

Step 9

- Receive the dental instrument from the operator and wipe it clean

Step 10

- Dispose of any waste material and waxed paper pad in the contaminated waste bin

Mixing time

- 30–60 seconds

Setting time

- 7–9 minutes

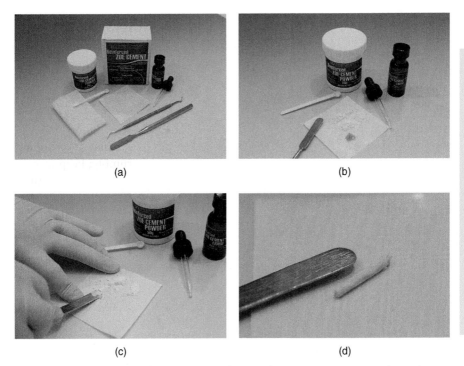

Figure 3.3 (a) ZOE set-up. (b) Step 3 – ZOE dispensed. (c) Step 6 – 'Stropping' during the mixing of ZOE. (d) Step 7 – ZOE final consistency as a temporary restorative material.

Instruments and materials used in set-up

- Waxed paper pad
- Broad-bladed spatula
- Zinc oxide eugenol powder and liquid, or capsule
- Flat plastic instrument

FURTHER READING

3M ESPE 2009: CAVIT^{TM} Material Safety Data Sheet. Available at http://multimedia. 3m.com/mws/mediawebserver?66666UtN&ZUxL99XlxfVO8TVOVu9KcuZgVU_LXT1u666666–pdf (Accessed: 10 April 2009).

Chapter 4
Non-aesthetic restorative materials

DENTAL AMALGAM

Definition

Dental amalgam is a permanent posterior restorative material that consists of silver alloy (silver, tin and copper) and mercury. Amalgam is supplied in encapsulated form and appears silver in the mouth. The mercury used within dental amalgam is a liquid metal (at room temperature) and is used to wet and bind the silver alloy once mixed. Once triturated with the metal, it forms a small, pliable material suitable for packing/condensing into the cavity preparation. Dental amalgam should always be used in conjunction with rubber dam to reduce the risk of inhalation in the event of accidental displacement (best practice). The mercury used in dental amalgam is minimal and should not pose a hazard to dental staff; however, care must be taken to not inhale the fumes, or have prolonged periods of skin contact, as this has been proven to be a health hazard (see *Special considerations for working with dental amalgam*).

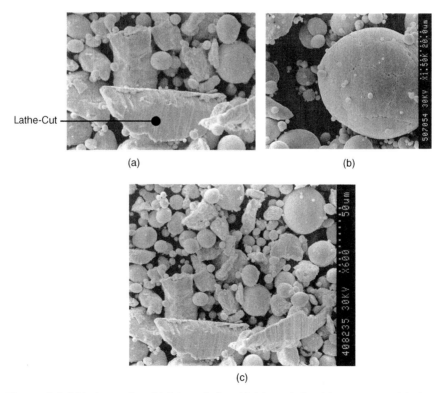

Lathe-Cut

(a)   (b)

(c)

Figure 4.1 (a) Lathe-cut alloy. (b) Spherical alloy. (c) Admixed alloy (photo courtesy of SDI).

Amalgam alloys are classified by their composition and particle shape. Lathe-cut alloy (Figure 4.1a) is made up or irregular-shaped alloy particles. Spherical alloy (Figure 4.1b) is made up of spherical shaped alloy particles and requires less mercury to bind the materials due to its smoothness. Admixed alloy (Figure 4.1c) is a mixture of both spherical and lathe-cut particles. Operators often choose a spherical or admixed alloy, as the spherical particles act as reinforcers and can be more closely packed, resulting in a higher strength amalgam. The amount of copper in amalgam classifies it as either a high- or low-copper amalgam. High-copper amalgams are preferred as they reduce the amount of corrosion and marginal breakdown in the oral cavity produced by the tin–mercury product gamma 2 ($\gamma2$) present in low-copper amalgams.

An **amalgam capsule** (Figure 4.2a) contains silver alloy, mercury, a mixing pestle and a plastic bubble (Figure 4.2b). The plastic bubble separates the

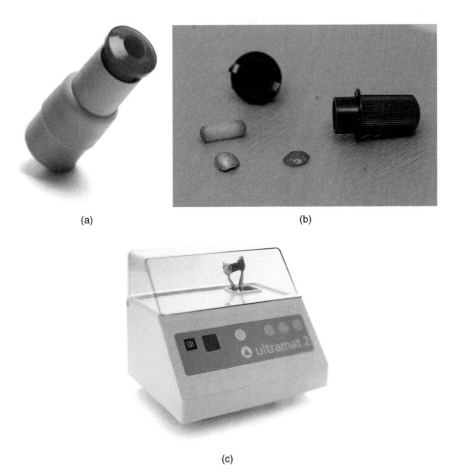

(a)　　　　(b)

(c)

Figure 4.2 (a) Amalgam capsule. (b) Amalgam capsule contents. (c) Amalgamator.

silver alloy and mercury until the user activates the capsule (depending on the manufacturer, the capsule may be squeezed, twisted or activated using a device supplied by the manufacturer). The function of the pestle is to mix the silver alloy and mercury together. Once the amalgam capsule is activated, it is placed in the amalgamator for trituration. **Trituration** is the process in which the amalgam capsule is shaken for a defined period of time and speed in order to mix the silver alloy and mercury to the desired consistency. The **amalgamator** (Figure 4.2c) triturates the capsule to uniformly mix the silver alloy and mercury, which results in a putty-like mix that can be manipulated and placed into the cavity preparation, allowing the operator sufficient time to condense (pack), carve and burnish (smooth) the material. The manufacturer's instructions should be followed in relation to the mixing time of the amalgam, as trituration time and speed may affect the properties of the amalgam.

Dental amalgam capsules contain '**spills**' of amalgam; a spill refers to the amount of material contained in the capsule. The capsules may be colour coded to help users distinguish between spills. Spills are referred to by numbers, i.e. 1 spill = a single mix (600 mg), 2 spills = a double mix (800 mg), etc. Three spill sizes are available (size may vary depending on the manufacturer). It is the operator that will request the spill of amalgam needed, which corresponds to the size of the cavity preparation to be filled. Amalgam may be purchased in bulk quantities or smaller ones (Figure 4.3).

An **amalgam waste container** (Figure 4.4) must be used to ensure safe and proper disposal of excess dental amalgam. Separate containers are available for

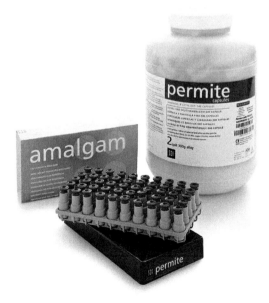

Figure 4.3 Amalgam packaging in bulk and small quantities.

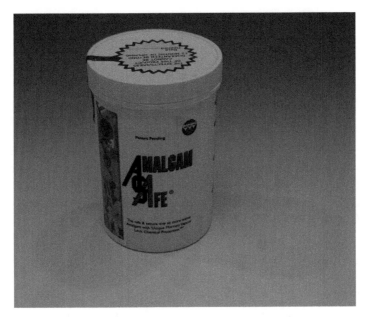

Figure 4.4 Amalgam waste container.

the excess amalgam and the amalgam capsule. The amalgam waste container is an airtight container that contains a foam insert containing non-hazardous chemicals (oxidising agent or activated charcoal) meant for suppressing mercury vapours.

Material constituents/composition

Silver alloy	Mercury
Silver	Mercury
Tin	
Copper	
(Sometimes zinc)	

Properties

- The strength of amalgam is dependent on the type of amalgam (spherical, high copper, etc.)

NON-AESTHETIC RESTORATIVE MATERIALS

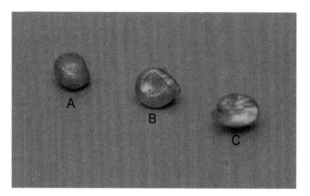

Figure 4.5 (a) Over-triturated amalgam. (b) Amalgam triturated to the correct timing. (c) Under-triturated amalgam.

- Amalgam reaches its final compressive strength after 24 hours (this may depend on amalgam types; e.g. a high-copper amalgam may reach its final compressive strength quicker)
- If occlusal forces are placed on amalgam too early post placement, there is a greater risk of fracture
- May be used in conjunction with a bonding agent to micromechanically adhere amalgam to the tooth and reduce the chances of microleakage
- May be used in conjunction with cavity varnish, liners and bases

Advantages

- Durable – able to withstand normal occlusal forces
- Low cost
- Easy to manipulate and place

Disadvantages

- Sensitive to mixing technique (incorrect trituration time of dental amalgam may affect the strength and dimensional change of the material) (Figure 4.5a, b and c)
- Undertriturated dental amalgam appears crumbly and dull
- Overtriturated amalgam appears sticky and wet
- Silver coloured

- Does not have bonding properties (if bonding is needed, the operator must use an appropriate bonding agent)

- Does not release fluoride

- Mercury is poisonous, therefore it must be handled and disposed of with great care

- Usually requires larger cavity preparation to provide sufficient mechanical retention

Indications and contraindications for use

Indications
- Permanent restorations in posterior teeth

- Core buildups

- Retrograde restorations (apicectomy)

Contraindications
- Mercury in amalgam requires precautions by the dental team to ensure their safety and the patient's safety during use

- Not suitable for restorations in anterior teeth due to silver colour

- Metallic properties pose the risk of thermal shock to the pulp and may require the use of liners, bases and/or varnishes

Trade names

Trade name	Manufacturer
Permite	SDI

Manipulation (Figures 4.6a–c)

Wearing personal protective equipment:

Step 1

- The tooth operator will administer local anaesthetic, if indicated

NON-AESTHETIC RESTORATIVE MATERIALS

- Tooth is appropriately prepared and isolated, and if liners, bases and bonding agents are needed, they are applied to cavity prior to amalgam placement

Step 2

- Activate the dental amalgam capsule (following the manufacturer's instructions); see Figure 4.2

Step 3

- Taking consideration to not cross-contaminate the amalgamator, load the activated amalgam capsule into the amalgamator. It is easier to load one end of the capsule first

- Close the cover of the amalgamator over the amalgam capsule (this cover is in place for the safety of the staff and patients in the event that the amalgam capsule becomes displaced from the amalgamator)

- The user can select the time for the amalgam to be triturated by dial or button (follow the manufacturer's instructions when selecting triturated time)

- To triturate the amalgam, the user must push the start button

- The amalgamator will stop automatically once the prescribed time has been reached

Step 4

- Remove the amalgam capsule from the amalgamator and open the capsule, carefully dropping contents into an amalgam well (precautions and care must be taken to not contact the contents of the amalgam capsule – if the pestle or bubble drop into the amalgam well, use college tweezers to remove and place into an empty amalgam capsule)

Step 5

- Using an amalgam carrier, collect amalgam material in increments for ease of placement by the operator (take care to wipe extra pieces of amalgam away that may drop while transferring the amalgam carrier to the operator)

- Pass the loaded amalgam carrier to the operator to place in the cavity preparation

- Be prepared to extend the amalgam plugger/condenser of choice to the operator and receive the amalgam carrier to refill

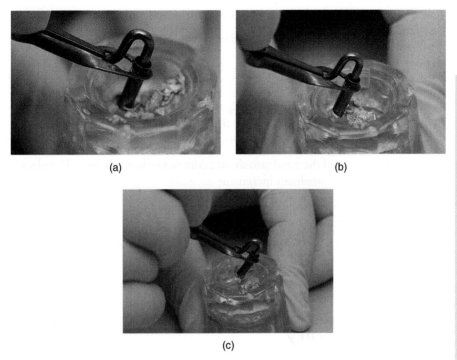

(a)   (b)

(c)

Figure 4.6 Filling amalgam carrier.

Step 6

- Repeat step 5 until the operator does not require any more amalgam

Step 7

- Ensure that the excess material is cleared from the working end of the amalgam carrier (to prevent amalgam setting in the amalgam carrier, rendering it unusable) and continue assisting the operator to condense, carve and burnish the restoration

Step 8

- At the completion of the treatment, care must be taken to dispose of excess amalgam material and amalgam capsule correctly in the amalgam waste container see Figure 4.4

- Dispose of the amalgam waste container with an authorized contractor

Mixing time

- Follow the manufacturer's instructions

- Overmixing amalgam causes contraction of the material
- Undermixing causes expansion of the material

Setting time

- Depends on the type of amalgam (the initial set takes place a few minutes after placement, and the final set takes many hours, up to 24 hours); there are fast and slow set types of amalgam available
- Condensing of the amalgam should commence immediately after placement of each amalgam increment
- Carving and burnishing of the amalgam can take place approximately three minutes after placement
- Finishing of amalgam should ideally take place 24 hours after placement

Special considerations for working with dental amalgam/mercury

- Always wear personal protective equipment – repeated contact with skin may allow mercury absorption, resulting in chronic mercury poisoning
- Jewellery may harbour loose amalgam particles and cause damage; therefore, jewellery should not be worn
- Never have direct contact with skin and dental amalgam (use the "no touch" technique)
- Work within a well-ventilated area
- Always use the high-volume evacuation/suction (and when removing amalgams use copious amounts of water) while working with dental amalgam (must be ventilated outside of the dental surgery)
- Always close the cover of the amalgamator over the amalgam capsule during use (this cover is in place for the safety of the operator in the event that the amalgam capsule becomes displaced from the amalgamator)
- Take care to dispose of all excess amalgam, including small particles in the amalgam waste container, or any similar airtight, non-breakable container – this container must be stored in a cool, ventilated area, as higher temperatures increase the amount of mercury vapour released
- Dispose of excess amalgam found in suction separators/traps (chair filters) as above

- Dispose of extracted teeth with amalgam fillings present as above

- Ensure that the waste amalgam container is disposed of properly by the appointed waste contractor – never dispose of in a waste bin

- In the event of a spill, follow the surgery policy to clean it up (see *Mercury spills*)

- Ensure all staff are aware of the presence, location and correct usage of the mercury spillage kit (see contents below)

- Ensure that during instrument clean-up all traces of amalgam are removed from instruments

Mercury spills

- In the event of a mercury spill, never attempt to clean it up with bare hands

- Open all windows to improve ventilation

- It is undesirable to have carpeted areas where amalgam is being used, as it is impossible to effectively clean mercury from a carpeted surface

- Many commercial products/kits are available to clean up mercury spills – ensure there is an office policy on how to clean up a mercury spill

- Contents of a mercury spill kit include variations of the following:

  o Gloves

  o Safety glasses and mask

  o Flowers of sulphur and calcium oxide

  o Brush

  o Syringe

- To clean up a small mercury spill, wear a mask, gloves and safety glasses

- Use the brush to bring all the spilled mercury together. Use the supplied syringe to draw up the loose mercury and dispose it of in the amalgam waste bin

- Use a mixture of flowers of sulphur, calcium oxide and water to cover the area where the spill occurred

- Once this mixture has dried on the surface, use wet disposable towels to clean up and dispose of all in the amalgam waste bin

- The amalgam waste bin needs to be disposed of appropriately after a spill

- All spills must be immediately reported to the dentist and recorded in the accident book

- If a large spill occurs, the local Health and Safety Authority (or equivalent in your area) must be informed. The American Dental Association (2003) recognises a large mercury spill as anything over 10 grams of mercury present

- A team meeting should take place to discuss the incident – how it was dealt with and how to prevent future accidents from occurring

Instruments and materials used in setup

The following instruments and materials used in setup:

- dental amalgam
- amalgamator

Optional:

- bonding agent

  o applicator brush
  o light-curing unit

- cavity varnish

  o applicator brush

- various bases and liners

  o spatula
  o applicator (instrument or brush)
  o paper pad
  o glass slab
  o light-curing unit

NB: When removing 'old' or existing amalgams, it is essential for the dental team to wear personal protective equipment (mask, gloves and glasses) and use copious amounts of water spray and high-volume suction.

Post-operative instructions to be given to the patient after the insertion of an amalgam restoration

- The patient should not eat for one hour and should eat on the opposite side of their mouth for 24 hours to allow the amalgam material to set. Occlusal forces on a newly inserted amalgam restoration may cause fracture

- Patients should be advised that the amalgam restoration may need to be polished on a return visit

- Patients should not consume anything too hot until the local anaesthetic has worn off to avoid burning themselves

- Patients need to be careful not to bite their lips and cheeks if local anaesthetic has been used, as this may be sore once sensation returns

REFERENCE

Journal of the American Dental Association (2003). Dental mercury hygiene recommendations. *Journal of the American Dental Associations*, *134*(11), 1498–1499. Available at http://jada.ada.org/cgi/content/abstract/134/11/1498 (Accessed: 10 April 2009).

NON-AESTHETIC RESTORATIVE MATERIALS

Chapter 5
Aesthetic restorative materials

There are many different types of aesthetically sound restorative materials available. The operator must choose the most suitable materials based on durability, cost, fluoride-releasing properties, aesthetics, chairside time and ease of use.

RESIN COMPOSITE

A resin composite material, by definition, is a material made from two or more substances (see *Composition* below). **Resin composite materials** have a number of clinical applications.

There are many types of resin composites on the market. The characteristics of some them are shown in the chart given below:

Dispensing options	Curing options	Flowability options
● Single use compule form (Figure 5.1a) ● Two-paste system (Figure 5.1b) ● Syringe form (Figure 5.1c and 5.1d)	● Dual cure ● Self-cure ● Light cure	● Flowable resin composites ● Packable/condensable resin composites ● Hybrid materials ● Nanofilled

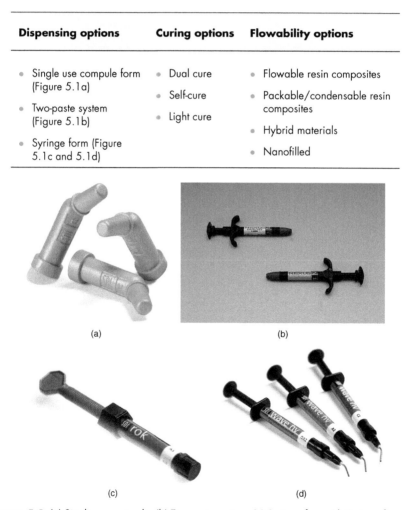

(a)   (b)

(c)   (d)

Figure 5.1 (a) Single-use compule. (b) Two-paste system. (c) Syringe form. (d) Syringe form.

Resin composites may be used in conjunction with acid etch, primers and bonding agents. The manufacturer's instructions for use should always be followed, as these may depend on each individual product.

Material constituents/composition

Resin composites consist of an organic resin, reinforcing filler and a coupling agent. The resin allows resin composite to be moulded and set by polymerisation (light or chemical curing); the filler contributes to the strength and hardness of the material; and the coupling agent binds the components together. Different types, sizes and shapes of fillers (powdered glass, quartz, ceramic particles and silica) affect the characteristics of individual resin composites.

There are various classifications of resin composite materials. Particle size varies between the types of resin composites. It can be classified into fine, microfill or a combination of both, which are referred to as 'hybrid' and, most recently, nanofilled.

Properties

- Strong

- Wear resistant

- Less durable than amalgam, but more aesthetically pleasing

- Used in conjunction with acid etch (phosphoric acid solution), primer and bonding agent

- Placed in increments with polymerisation (light curing) in between to ensure the curing of all layers and to reduce the opportunity for shrinkage

- Less dense than amalgam

Advantages

- Aesthetically pleasing

- Working time of light-cured resin composite can be operator controlled

- Strong

- Mechanically bonds to the tooth structure

- Operator can be conservative during restorations (due to mechanical bond)

AESTHETIC RESTORATIVE MATERIALS

Disadvantages

- It is not condensable or packable (this includes posterior composite materials in the true sense of packable)
- Technique sensitive (follow the manufacture's instructions for specific product specifications and usage)
- Shrinkage upon polymerisation
- Time consuming (takes approximately three times longer than placing an amalgam restoration of comparable size)
- Does not release fluoride
- Moisture intolerant
- Tends to 'stick' to dental instruments; may require use of special dental instruments

Indications and contraindications for use

Indications
- Permanent restorations – especially on anterior teeth
- Core buildups
- Temporary/provisional restorations
- Direct veneers
- Class I, Class II, Class III, Class IV and Class V restorations
- Specially formulated resin composite materials are available for Class II posterior applications

Contraindications
- Not to be used with cavity varnish (prevents adhesion)
- Unsuitable for use where it may be difficult to maintain good moisture control
- Patients with grinding (bruxism) habits
- Replacement of posterior cusps (due to high load, which increases risk of wear and fracture on resin composite)
- Large restorations on posterior teeth (the larger the restoration, the greater the polymerisation shrinkage)
- Deep restorations extending subgingivally (difficult to achieve good marginal seal and effective moisture control)

Trade names

Trade name	Manufacturer	Usage
EsthetX *Flow*®	Dentsply	Flowable resin composite
Filtek™ Supreme	3M ESPE	Nanofilled
Glacier (Figure 5.2a)	SDI	Anterior and posterior restorations
Herculite® (Figure 5.2b)	Kerr	Small particle hybrid (anterior and posterior restorations)
Ice	SDI	Various usages
Integrity™	Dentsply	Temporary/provisional restorations
P60™	3M ESPE	Packable/condensable resin composite
Revolution™ (Figure 5.2c)	Kerr	Flowable resin composite
Rock	SDI	Posterior restorations
Surefil™	Dentsply	Packable/condensable resin composite
Tetric	Ivoclar	Different types available for different usages
Wave (Figure 5.2d)	SDI	Flowable resin composite

AESTHETIC RESTORATIVE MATERIALS

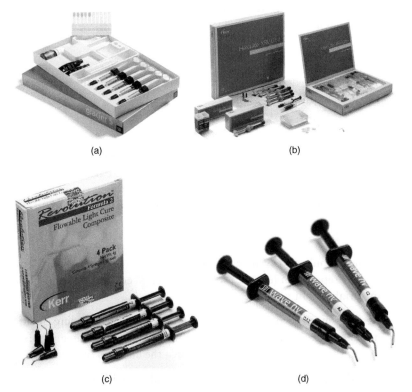

(a)

(b)

(c)

(d)

Figure 5.2 (a) Glacier – SDI. (b) Herculite® – Kerr. (c) Revolution™ – Kerr. (d) Wave – SDI.

Manipulation (Figures 5.3a–5.3c)

Wearing personal protective equipment:

Follow the manufacturer's instructions for storage of resin composite material. Most products are best stored in the refrigerator and brought to room temperature prior to use.

Step 1

- The operator will administer local anaesthetic, if indicated
- Pass the operator the shade guide for shade selection (using a natural light source) of the tooth/teeth being treated (prior to drying of the teeth)
- Tooth is appropriately prepared and isolated, and if liners, bases and bonding agents are needed, they are applied prior to resin composite placement

Step 2

- Prepare the tooth for resin composite placement using operator's choice of acid etchant and bonding system (see Chapter 6)

Step 3

- The choice of delivery system for resin composite will determine dispensing instructions

Two-paste system

- If using the two-paste system, dispense equal lengths of both the catalyst and base on the waxed paper pad, taking care that they do not touch. When requested, mix them together (mixing time: 30 seconds) with a plastic mixing spatula until a uniform colour is reached

Compule and syringe type

- Both compule and syringe type resin composites can be added directly to the preparation (ensure the cap(s) is replaced after placement, as the material is light sensitive)
- Resin composite may be added directly over the bonding agent and needs to be added incrementally (2mm) to ensure complete polymerisation of each increment and to reduce the chances of shrinkage
- Pass the resin composite to the operator along with a Teflon-tipped flat plastic instrument

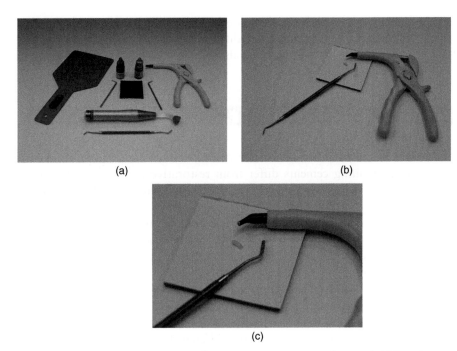

(a)

(b)

(c)

Figure 5.3 (a) Resin composite set-up. (b) Step 3 – resin composite dispensed. (c) Step 4 –
resin composite ready for transfer to the operator.

Step 4

- Repeat step 4 until the operator has enough resin composites. Be prepared with gauze to wipe the blunt dental instrument in between applications

Step 5

- Dispose of the paper mixing pad and the remaining resin composite
  (left on the paper mixing pad or the resin composite compule and the
  disposable applicator brush in the contaminated waste)

Mixing time

- Two-paste system: 30 seconds

Setting time

- Two-paste system – setting begins immediately (dual cure) or it may
  be polymerised for 30 seconds

- Light cured – minimum 40 seconds per 2-millimetre depth (follow the manufacturer's instructions as different products and light-curing units will require a variation on the above)

GLASS IONOMER

Glass ionomer may be used as a restorative material, a liner or a luting agent. Glass ionomer luting cements differ from restorative materials by having a smaller particle size. In this chapter, they will be discussed in the context of **luting cements.**

Glass ionomers, which are a diverse group of materials, are supplied in many different forms. It is the particle size of a glass ionomer that dictates its usage. Luting and lining materials have smaller particle sizes than restorative forms of glass ionomer.

Glass ionomer cements have three main characteristics; the ability to release fluoride, they can chemically bond to dentine, and they can be added to the preparation in bulk (there is no need for incremental placement).

Glass ionomers are supplied in many different forms and can be classified as follows:

Type I Glass Ionomer: Luting cement (crown and bridge)
Type II Glass Ionomer: Class V and III restorations (aesthetic)
Type III Glass Ionomer: Liner or base (opaque)
Type IV Glass Ionomer: Crown and core build-up.

Material constituents/composition

Supplied in:

- Pre-measured, pre-capsulated form (needs activation and trituration)
- Powder and liquid form

Powder and liquid constituents:

Powder	Liquid
• Aluminosilicate glass particles – (these can vary in size to give each type of material its different characteristics)	• Polyalkenoic acid in water • Some materials include Tartaric acid / malric acid

Properties

- Highest release of fluoride of all restorative materials
- Not as durable as many other materials, high wear rate and can be brittle
- Chemically bonds to enamel, dentine and some alloys, e.g. tin-plated crown
- Aesthetics inferior to resin composite material
- Moisture sensitive – both to excessive wetting and excessive drying
- May be used in conjunction with a conditioner to remove the dentinal smear layer where appropriate
- May require a plastic spatula for manipulation; check the manufacturer's instructions

Advantages

- Bonds directly to enamel and dentine
- Does not need to be applied incrementally
- Releases fluoride
- Can be set by polymerisation

Disadvantages

- Mixing glass ionomer material is technique sensitive, and the correct liquid / powder ratio must be used (cement will become weaker with incorrect mixing proportions). Capsulated mixes are preferred for this reason
- Short working time
- Long setting time
- Moisture sensitive
- Brittle material
- Translucency of glass ionomer is inferior to resin composite
- Not as strong as amalgam or resin composites
- Type II requires a minimum of 15 minutes prior to polishing and may need a surface coat (manufacturers supply varnish or clear resin)

AESTHETIC RESTORATIVE MATERIALS

Indications and contraindications for use

Indications for glass ionomers vary depending on its composition. The dental team must choose a product dependent on its intended purpose. (There is not one product that is suitable for all indicated clinical situations.)

Indications

- Occlusal restorations in primary teeth
- Bases and liners
- Proximal lesions
- Temporary restorations
- Cervical lesions
- Repair of crown margins
- Abrasion and erosion lesions
- Core buildups
- Luting cement – crowns, bridges and inlays
- Class III restorations
- May be used in conjunction with calcium hydroxide in the event of pulpal exposure

Contraindications

- In areas of extensive occlusal caries
- In areas where there would be strong occlusal forces (e.g. incisal tips, cusps and pin-retained cores)

Trade names

Trade name	Manufacturer
Ketac™-fil	3M ESPE
Ketac™-Molar	3M ESPE
Riva Self Cure capsulated form (Figure 5.4a)	SDI
Riva Self Powder/liquid form (Figure 5.4b)	SDI

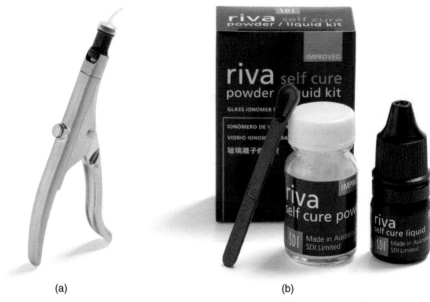

(a) (b)

Figure 5.4 (a) Riva self-cure capsulated form – SDI. (b) Riva self-cure powder and liquid – SDI.

Manipulation (restorative material)

See manipulation under *Resin-modified glass ionomer*.

Mixing time

- Depends on the type of material used and its clinical indication

Setting time

- 3–6 minutes depending on the type and use of the glass ionomer material
- Type II – coat surface immediately with varnish (supplied by manufacturer or clear resin) on initial set

RESIN-MODIFIED GLASS IONOMER

A resin modified glass ionomer is a glass ionomer with resin composite properties. It contains a resin (like a resin composite) that allows it to be set with a curing light (this is opposite to a compomer which is a resin composite with glass ionomer properties). Resin-modified glass ionomers are most often used for restorations in non-stress-bearing areas in patients with a high risk of caries.

Material constituents/composition

Powder and liquid constituents:

Powder	Liquid
Fluoro-aluminosilicate glass	Acidic resin
	Primer resin

Properties

- Releases fluoride (greater than resin composite and compomers, but less than glass ionomers)
- Easily manipulated
- Polymerised

Advantages

- Setting time can be reduced with polymerisation
- Aesthetic appearance
- Prolonged working time in comparison to glass ionomer
- Bonds directly to enamel and dentine (often used in conjunction with conditioner of 10–20% polyacrylic acid for 10 seconds)
- Releases fluoride (greater than resin composite and compomers, but less than glass ionomers)
- There is a fluoride recharge when exposed to fluoride sources (e.g. topical fluoride and fluoride toothpaste)
- Can be polished and finished immediately
- If used in conjunction with resin composite, a bond is formed (no need to etch surface)

AESTHETIC RESTORATIVE MATERIALS

Disadvantages

- Shrinkage due to polymerisation
- Incremental addition of the material needed due to polymerisation

Indications and contraindications for use

Indications for resin-modified glass ionomers vary depending on their composition. The dental team must choose a product depending on its intended purpose. (There is not one product that is suitable for all indicated clinical uses.)

Indications
- Posterior restorations in primary teeth
- Class III restorations
- Class V restorations
- Crown and bridge luting cement
- Base and liner

Contraindications
- Occlusal and Class II restorations
- Allergy to resin component
- Use in high-stress areas or areas where there are heavy masicatory forces
- Should not be used in conjunction with a bonding agent, as it will decrease the fluoride release

Trade names

Trade name	Manufacturer
Fuji II LC (type 2) – capsulated form (Figure 5.5a)	GC America
Fuji II LC (type 2) – powder / liquid form (Figure 5.5b)	GC America
Photac™ Fil (type 2)	3M ESPE
Vitremer™ (type 2)	3M ESPE

AESTHETIC RESTORATIVE MATERIALS

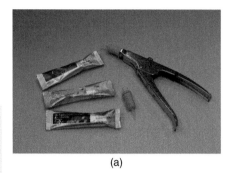 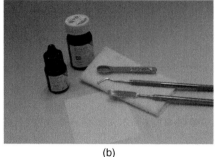

(a)   (b)

Figure 5.5 (a) Fuji II capsulated form – 3M ESPE. (b) Fuji II powder and liquid – 3M ESPE.

Manipulation (Figures 5.6a–c and 5.7)

Wearing personal protective equipment:

Step 1

- The operator will administer local anaesthetic, if indicated
- Tooth is appropriately prepared and isolated, and if liners, bases and bonding agents are needed, they are applied prior to placement

Step 2

- Apply conditioner (10–20% polyacrylic acid for 10 seconds) to the dentine to remove the smear layer

Step 3

- Rinse and gently dry the area with a cotton pellet

Step 4
Powder and liquid form:

- Fluff powder by shaking, ensuring caps are on tight
- Dispense material (measure level scoops and accurately drop liquid)
- Recap powder and liquid

Capsulated form (Figure 5.7):

- Activate the capsule (following the manufacturer's instructions)

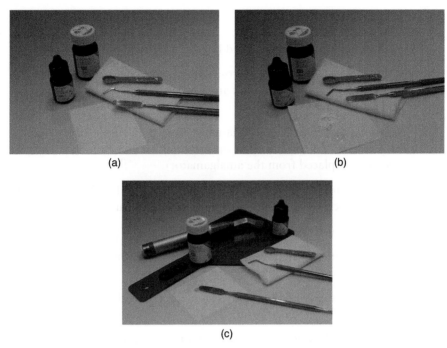

Figure 5.6 (a) Resin-modified glass ionomer set-up. (b) Step 4 – resin-modified glass ionomer dispensed. (c) Step 5 – resin-modified glass ionomer mixed.

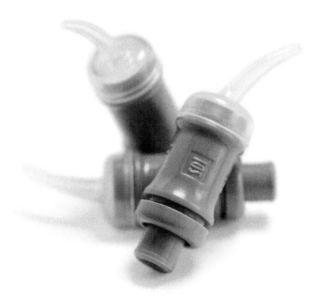

Figure 5.7 Resin-modified glass ionomer capsule.

Step 5

- Skip step 5 if using powder and liquid form of material
- Taking consideration to not cross-contaminate the amalgamator, load the activated capsule into the amalgamator. It is easiest to load one end of the capsule first
- Close the cover of the amalgamator over the capsule (this cover is in place for the safety of the operator in the event that the capsule becomes displaced from the amalgamator)
- The user can select the time for trituration by dial or button (follow the manufacturer's instructions when selecting trituration time)
- User must push the start button
- The amalgamator will stop automatically once the desired time has been reached
- Remove the capsule from the amalgamator and load into the dispensing gun supplied by the manufacturer
- *Skip step 6 if using capsulated form of resin modified glass ionomer material*

Step 6

- Mix the powder and liquid using a Weston spatula or plastic spatula (if indicated by the manufacturer) until a homogenous (even) mixture has been achieved – the mixture should appear glossy
- Powder and liquid must be incorporated in two increments, follow the manufacturer's instructions for mixing time

Step 7

- Pass the operator the material on waxed paper pad along with plastic instrument for placement
- Be prepared with gauze to wipe the blunt instrument for the operator

Step 8

- Light cure material, as indicated by the manufacturer's instructions

Step 9

- Dispose of waxed paper pad, capsule (if used) and excess material in the contaminated waste

Mixing time

- Depends on the type of material used and its clinical indication

Setting time

- The material will slowly start to set once mixed (it will take 15–20 minutes without light curing, but can be light cured and set in 30 seconds)

COMPOMER (POLYACID-MODIFIED RESIN COMPOSITE)

A compomer is a material that combines the properties of resin composites and glass ionomers. It is virtually a resin composite that has been modified to incorporate some of the fluoride-releasing properties of a glass ionomer. (This is the opposite of a resin-modified glass ionomer, which is a glass ionomer with resin-composite properties.)

Material constituents/composition

Supplied in compules or syringes:

- Hydrophilic monomers
- Fluoro-aluminosilicate glass
- Dimethacrylate monomer
- Special resin
- Photoactivators/initiators

Properties

- Fluoride release (lower amount of fluoride release than glass ionomers)
- Fluoride release varies from product to product

- Mechanical properties and wear resistance is inferior to resin composites, but superior to glass ionomers

Indications and contraindications for use

Indications

- Restorations in primary teeth

- Restorations in low stress-bearing areas

- Class III restorations

- Class IV restorations

- Long-term temporary restorations

- Luting

Contraindications

- Lacks the ability to directly adhere chemically to any tooth surface

- Moisture sensitive

- Technique sensitive

- Not for use in high-stress areas

Trade names

Trade name	Manufacturer
Compoglass	Ivoclar
Dyract® Ap	Dentsply
F2000™	3M ESPE

Manipulation

Wearing personal protective equipment:

Step 1

- The operator will administer local anaesthetic, if indicated

- Pass the operator the shade guide for shade selection of the tooth/teeth being treated (prior to drying of the teeth)

- Tooth is appropriately prepared and isolated, and if liners, bases and bonding agents are needed, they are applied prior to compomer placement

Step 2

- Prior to application of the compomer material, the operator will apply an acid etchant/bonding system of his or her choice (see Chapter 6)

Step 3

- Compomer can be added directly to the preparation, ensuring that the cap is replaced after placement, as the material is light sensitive

- Compomer may be added directly over the bonding agent, and most often needs to be added incrementally to ensure complete curing and to reduce the opportunity for shrinkage. Each increment is individually light cured

- Pass the compomer material to the operator along with a Teflon-tipped, flat plastic instrument

Step 4

- Repeat step 3 until the operator has enough compomer

- Have gauze ready to wipe instrument between applications

Step 5

- Dispose of waxed paper pad, remaining compomer (left on pad or compomer compule) and disposable applicator brush in the contaminated waste

Mixing time

- Distributed in compules or syringes – no mixing required

Setting time

- Light cured – normally minimum 40 seconds per 2-millimetre depth (follow the manufacturer's instructions)

Instruments and materials used in set-up

Materials used in set-up:

- restorative materials

- ○ waxed paper pad
- ○ dispensing gun (if using compules)
- • Primer and bonding agent (if material indicates use)
- ○ acid etch (if indicated)
- ○ disposable applicator brush
- ○ dispensing well for bonding agent, with amber shield to protect from light

FURTHER READING

van Noort, R. (2007). *Introduction to Dental Materials*, 3rd edn. London: Elsevier.

Chapter 6
Acid etchant, bonding agents and fissure sealants

ACID ETCHANT

Definition

Acid etchant (more commonly known as acid etch) is available in a phosphoric acid solution or gel and is commonly available in 15%, 34% or 37% concentrations (37% being the most common). Acid etch creates microscopic spaces in enamel (increasing surface roughness) into which the bonding agent/adhesive can flow, aiding the bonding process (micromechanical retention). When desiccated, a surface that has been etched appears chalky white or frosted (Figure 6.1c). Acid etch also removes contaminants from the surface, aiding in the wettability of the enamel. (It removes the smear layer and acquired pellicle.)

An acid is used to remove some of the mineral elements in the tooth to promote adhesion. When placing a restoration into a cavity preparation (Figure 6.1a), it is usually desirable or essential (when working with certain materials) to use an acid etch (Figure 6.1b) and resin adhesive to adhere/bond the restoration to the tooth structure (enamel or dentine).

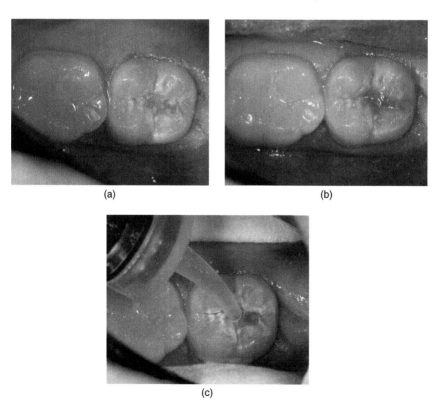

(a)   (b)

(c)

Figure 6.1 (a) Prepared tooth surface prior to acid etchant placement. (b) Acid etchant placement. (c) Chalky white/frosted appearance of acid etchant (photos courtesy of Dr. Mitsuru).

Material constituents/composition

- Phosphoric acid solution
  Available in:
  - liquid solution (rarely used)
  - gel (tends to be easier to use as it does not run)
  - syringes or bottles

Properties

- Moisture sensitive
- Best practice is to use a rubber dam when using acid etch
- Prior to use, the surface must be clean (use pumice and brush – do not use prophylaxis paste as the fluoride and other constituents may leave residue and interfere with bonding properties)

Advantages

- Creates a surface roughness of enamel that aids in increasing the wettability of enamel, which allows for the micromechanical bond between the restorative material and enamel

Disadvantages

- Care must be taken to protect eyes, skin and intra-oral soft tissues when using acid etch due to its acidic properties. The dental team should always wear appropriate personal protective equipment, as well as ensuring the patient wears protective eye wear
- Technique sensitive

Indications and contraindications for use

Indications
- In areas where a micromechanical bond is desired, such as sealant placement, resin composite restorations, directly bonded orthodontic brackets, veneers and resin-bonded crowns and bridges

ACID ETCHANT, BONDING AGENTS AND FISSURE SEALANTS

Contraindications

- May be difficult to use in children, patients with special needs and the elderly as it may be hard to achieve good moisture control

- Should not be used in patients where excellent moisture control is not possible

- Should not be used during treatment of patients who cannot tolerate or facilitate time-consuming appointments

Trade names

Trade name	Manufacturer
Gel Etchant (Figure 6.2a)	Kerr
Microdose Etch (Figure 6.2b)	Premier
Super Etch (Figure 6.2c)	SDI
Total Etch	Ivoclar

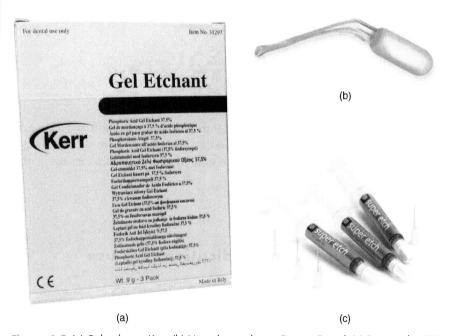

Figure 6.2 (a) Gel etchant – Kerr. (b) Microdose etchant – Premier Dental. (c) Super etch – SDI.

Manipulation

See below – manipulation for acid etch and bonding agents are combined as they are often used in conjunction with each other.

Mixing time
- There is no mixing with acid etch – it comes ready for use

DENTINE PRIMER AND BONDING AGENT

Dentine primer or dentinal conditioner may be used at the operator's discretion, following the manufacturer's instructions, after acid etching. The purpose of adding a dental primer is to wet the dentine and penetrate into the dentinal tubules as enamel-bonding agents cannot penetrate dentine.

A **bonding agent** (also referred to as adhesive) is often used in conjunction with acid etch. It aids in the retention between the restorative material and the tooth; it also fills the microscopic space that is left between a restoration and the tooth structure. Filling this space is beneficial as it reduces the chance of microleakage around the restoration. The bonding agent may directly adhere to the enamel, or to the primer used with exposed dentine.

There are many **bonding or adhesive** systems on the market, which include all the materials that are normally needed during the bonding process.

Material constituents/composition

- Primer (dentine conditioner) – soaks into the enamel and dentine

  - Seals dentine tubules

  - Forms a hybrid layer

- Adhesive/bond – joins hybrid to composite

Properties

- Using a bonding agent in conjunction with acid etch can decrease temperature sensitivity experienced by the patient

- Dentine/enamel bonding systems classification: (van Meerbeek, 2003)

  - Etch and rinse
    3 bottle
    o Etchant

  - o Primer – primer is dissolved in various solutions (e.g. acetone, alcohol or water), which requires it to be directly applied to a single-use applicator brush (disposable)
  - o Adhesive/bond
  - *2 bottle*
  - o Etchant
  - o Primer/adhesive/bond – primer is dissolved in various solutions (e.g. acetone, alcohol or water), which requires it to be directly applied to a single-use applicator brush (disposable)

- Self-etching – non-rinse
  2 bottle (no separate etch)
  - o Acidic primer
  - o Adhesive/bond
  1 bottle (all-in-one)
  - o Contains all

Advantages

- Enables the usage of resin-based products by promoting adhesion to tooth structures

Disadvantages

- Dentine is hydrophilic (water loving) and bonding agents are hydrophobic (water hating)

Indications and contraindications for use

Indications
- Bonding agents are suitable for use with amalgam, composites, compomer, resin-modified glass ionomers, porcelain, resins and precious and non-precious metals
- Bonding agents are used in conjunction with the cementation of orthodontic brackets, veneers, porcelain crowns and bridges

Contraindications
- Not indicated for use where there are pulpal exposures or saliva or blood contamination

Trade names

Adper™ Easy Bond Self-Etch Adhesive (3M ESPE)	Self-etch, all-in-one
Adper™ Prompt L-Pop (3M ESPE)	Self-etch, all-in-one
All-bond 2 (Bisco)	Etch and rinse, 3 bottle
Frog (SDI) (Figure 6.3a)	Self-etch, 2 bottle
Go! (SDI) (bottle – Figure 6.3b) (single dose – Figure 6.3c)	Self-etch, 1 bottle
Optibond Solo Plus (Kerr) (Figure 6.3d)	Etch and rinse, 2 bottle
One-step Plus (Bisco)	Etch and rinse, 2 bottle
OptiBond Solo Plus (Kerr)	Self-etch, 2 bottle

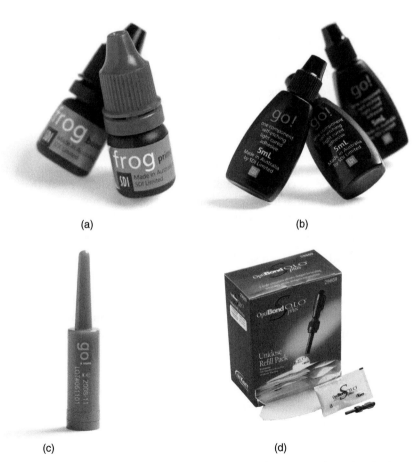

(a)   (b)

(c)   (d)

Figure 6.3 (a) Frog – SDI. (b) Go! bottle – SDI. (c) Go! uni dose – SDI. (d) Optibond Solo Plus – Kerr.

ACID ETCHANT, BONDING AGENTS AND FISSURE SEALANTS

Manipulation (acid etchant, primer and bonding agent) (Figures 6.4a–6.4g)

Wearing personal protective equipment:

Step 1

- Isolate, prepare and clean the tooth/teeth to be treated

Step 2

- The operator will add a dental liner where appropriate

Step 3

- Rinse with water and dry the tooth

  Skip steps 4, 5 and 6 if using etch and rinse – 2 bottle, self-etching – 2 bottle or self-etching – 1 bottle.

Step 4

- Dental nurse will prepare acid etch for dispensing

  - Syringe – expel a small amount of acid etch prior to handing to the operator to ensure there are no air bubbles, etc. present that may result in the acid etch being placed where it is not wanted (ensure syringe tip is replaced with a new one for each patient and disposed of in the sharps container – syringe tip is a single-use item)

  - Liquid – dispense a small amount of liquid into a dispensing well and hand it to the operator together with a disposable applicator brush

  - **Care needs to be taken during the handling and passing of acid etch as, if improperly handled, it can cause a health and safety risk to the dental team**

Step 5

- Pass acid etch to the operator who will apply it for 15–30 seconds (30 seconds on enamel, 15 seconds on dentine) (follow the manufacturer's instructions)

Step 6

- Rinse thoroughly for at least 20 seconds (using high-volume suction for evacuation to prevent acid etchant coming in contact with soft tissues as this can cause irritation) and gently dry the surface with damp cotton pellet to ensure the surface is not desiccated

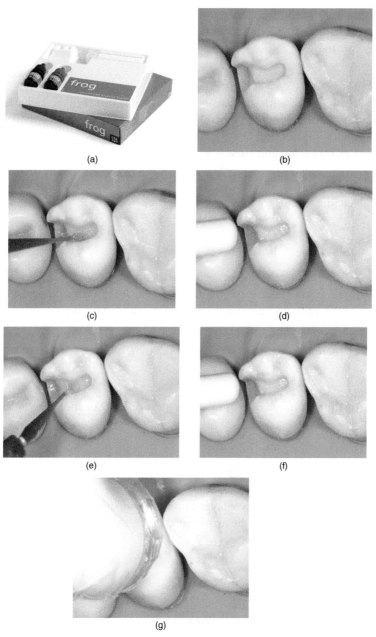

(a)   (b)   (c)   (d)   (e)   (f)   (g)

Figure 6.4 (a) Self-etch, 2 bottle set-up. The photos (b)–(g) depict the application of Frog – self-etch, 2 bottle-bonding system, refer to manipulation instructions for use of other dentine/enamel bonding systems (photos courtesy of Dr. Geoff Knight). (b) Step 1 – tooth prepared and isolated. (c) Step 2 – application of acidic primer (leave on surface for 20 seconds). (d) Step 7 – air dry for a minimum of 9 seconds (tooth does not require the addition of liners, and the Frog system is self-etch, 2 bottle, which does not require the application of a separate acid etchant). (e) Step 7 – application of adhesive/bond. (f) Step 7 – air dry for a minimum of 9 seconds. (g) Step 8 – polymerise for 10 seconds.

- It is very important that good isolation is maintained as any moisture will contaminate the surface, requiring the etching procedure to be repeated

Step 7

- Be prepared with dispensing well, applicator brush, light curing unit (if using bond/adhesive), amber eye protection shield (if using bond/adhesive) and one of the following materials:

  primer (etch and rinse – 3 bottle)

  primer/adhesive (etch and rinse – 2 bottle)

  acidic primer (self-etching – 2 bottle)

  or

  all-in-one (self-etching – 1 bottle)

- NB: Primer (etch and rinse 3 bottle) and primer/adhesive (etch and rinse 2 bottle) is dissolved in acetone, which requires it to be dispensed directly onto a single-use applicator brush (disposable)
- Leave on the surface for 20 seconds – following the manufacturer's instructions for the application of the material

Step 8

- Air thin using the 3-in-1/air-water syringe for 9 or more seconds
- **If using:**

  etch and rinse – 3 bottle

  self-etching – 2 bottle

  The primer has been air-thinned, and now the adhesive layer must be added. Add the adhesive layer using a new disposable applicator brush. This layer must also be air-thinned using the 3-in-1/air-water syringe for 9 or more seconds.
- **If using:**

  etch and rinse – 2 bottle

  self-etching – 1 bottle

  The adhesive has been air-thinned.

Step 9 (Follow the manufacturer's instructions in relation to material poly-merisation)

- Using the curing light and amber light protection shield, polymerise the layer of bonding agent for 10 seconds (following the manufacturer's instructions)

- If desired, repeat by adding another layer of bonding/adhesive, air-thin and polymerise (follow the manufacturer's instructions)

Step 10

- Continue the procedure as indicated by the treatment being provided

Step 11

- Wipe excess acid etch, primer and bonding agent from all surfaces using gauze with care (no-touch technique) and along with disposable brushes, dispose of in the contaminated waste

Instruments and materials used in set-up

- Choice of dentine/enamel bonding system
- Acid etchant (if required)
- Disposable applicator brushes
- Dispensing well, with amber cover to protect from light
- Light curing unit and amber light protection shield
- A three-in-one syringe/air-water syringe

ACID ETCHANT, BONDING AGENTS
AND FISSURE SEALANTS

FISSURE SEALANTS

Definition

Fissure sealants (Figure 6.5) are either resin composites or glass ionomers that are most often applied to occlusal pits and fissures of permanent posterior teeth. The anatomy of the occlusal surfaces of posterior permanent teeth makes them bacteria traps that are hard to clean, possibly leaving them susceptible to caries. Fissure sealants are used to create a smooth surface that is easily cleaned over the pits and fissures. Fissure sealants are a preventative measure indicated in patients with a history of caries or who are considered to be at high risk of caries. Consult the British Society of Paediatric Dentistry (2000) for more information in relation to indications of fissure sealants.

Material constituents/composition

- BIS-GMA (Bisphenol A-glycidyl methacrylate)
- Polymer
- Sealant may have added fillers for increased strength and hardness

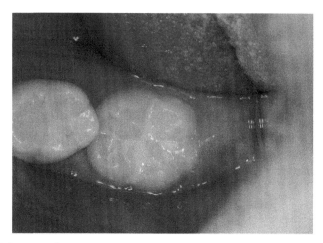

Figure 6.5 Fissure sealant.

Fissure sealant material is available in syringe form or in a bottle.

Properties

- Fissure sealant material must be of a low enough viscosity to flow easily
- Teeth must be thoroughly cleaned, etched and dried prior to application
- Fissure sealant material may be used in conjunction with bonding/adhesives

Advantages

- Mechanical bonding to enamel

Disadvantages

- Technique sensitive (must maintain a clear and dry working field)
- Moisture sensitive
- Must be monitored for microleakage, as this may result in failure of the fissure sealant

Indications and contraindications for use

Indications
- Indicated in patients with a history of caries or those that are at risk of caries
- Most often placed in children and young adults in pits and fissures to prevent bacteria entering this area

- Consult the British Society of Paediatric Dentistry's *Fissure sealants in paediatric dentistry: a policy document* for more indications of applications of fissure sealants

Contraindications
- In areas of exposed dentine
- Do not use prophylaxis paste to clean area prior to fissure sealant application as the fluoride content will inhibit bonding to the enamel

Trade names

Trade name	Manufacturer
Clinpro™ Sealant	3M ESPE
Conseal F bottle (Figure 6.6a)	SDI
Conseal F syringe (Figure 6.6b)	SDI
Flurosheild™	Dentsply
Helioseal (Figure 6.6c)	Vivadent
Seal-Rite™ (Figure 6.6d)	Pulpdent

ACID ETCHANT, BONDING AGENTS
AND FISSURE SEALANTS

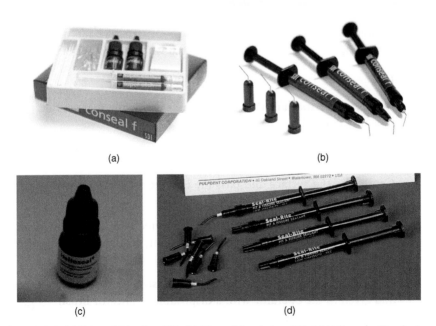

(a)　　　　　　　　　　　　　　　(b)

(c)　　　　　　　　　　　　　　　(d)

Figure 6.6 (a) Conseal F bottle – SDI. (b) Conseal F syringe – SDI. (c) Helioseal – Vivadent. (d) Sealrite – Pulpdent.

Manipulation (Figure 6.4)

Wearing personal protective equipment:

Step1

- The enamel surface of the tooth to be treated is cleaned with a mixture of pumice and water and rinsed and dried with an air-water syringe or a 3-in-1 syringe

Step 2

- Isolate the tooth/teeth to be fissure sealed effectively using cotton wool rolls and high-volume suction (moisture control is very important). If there is saliva contamination, the bonding process may be ineffective and the procedure may have to be repeated

Step 3

- Pass the acid etch to the operator for application. The acid etch is applied to the tooth surface for 15–30 seconds (following the manufacturer's instructions). Next, thoroughly wash and gently dry the tooth using both the 3-in-1 syringe/air-water syringe and the high-volume suction
- Acid etch creates microscopic spaces in the tooth tissue, which aids in bonding the fissure sealant to the tooth structure (an acid-etched surface appears 'chalky white' or frosted when desiccated)

Step 4

- Re-isolate the tooth/teeth to be fissure-sealed while maintaining good moisture control

Step 5

- Gently dry the surface and pass the operator the sealant material for application
- Syringe type fissure sealant can be added directly to the etched enamel (ensure the cap is replaced after placement, as the material is light-sensitive)
- Bottle types of fissure sealant need to be dispensed into a dappen dish and given to the operator with a disposable applicator brush
- Ensure the high-volume suction is ready to evacuate any moisture to avoid saliva contamination of the area

Step 6

- Polymerise the sealant material for a minimum of 40 seconds using a curing light (follow the manufacturer's instructions)

Step 7

- Pass the contra angled sickle probe and Millers forceps to the operator to check fissure sealant placement and occlusion

Step 8

- Dispose of excess material, disposable applicator brush and/or tip of the sealant syringe in the contaminated waste bin

Mixing time

- No mixing required

Setting time

- Polymerised

ACID ETCHANT, BONDING AGENTS AND FISSURE SEALANTS

Instruments and materials used in set-up (Figure 6.7)

- Pumice and water mixture
- Acid etchant
- Sealant material
- Applicator brush or disposal tip for sealant syringe
- Dappen dish
- Curing light
- Amber light protection shield
- Cotton wool rolls
- Cotton pellets

ACID ETCHANT, BONDING AGENTS
AND FISSURE SEALANTS

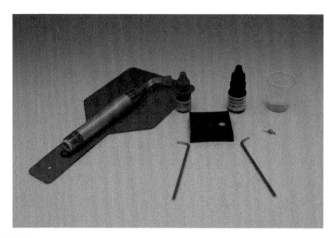

Figure 6.7 Sealant set-up.

FURTHER READING

British Society of Paediatric Dentistry (2000). Fissure sealants in paediatric dentistry: a policy document. *International Journal of Paediatric Dentistry* 10:174–177.

Kugal, G. (2000). The science of bonding: from first to sixth generation. *Journal of the American Dental Association*; 131:20–25.

Ripa, L.W., Wolff M.S. (1992). Preventive resin restorations: indications, technique, and success. *Quintessence International*; 23(5):307–315.

Van Meerbeek, B., De Munck, J., Yoshida, Y., Inoue, S., Vargas, M., Vijay, P., Van Landuyt, K., Lambrechts, P. and Vanherle, G. (2003). Buonocore memorial lecture. Adhesion to enamel and dentin: current status and future challenges. *Operative Dentistry*; 28:215–235.

Chapter 7
Liner and bases

Intermediate restorative materials are materials that are placed between a restoration and the dentine with a primary function of protecting the pulp. Dental liners, bases and cavity varnishes are used for this purpose.

A **dental liner** is a material that is usually placed in a thin layer over exposed dentine within a cavity preparation. Its functions are dentinal sealing, pulpal protection, thermal insulation and stimulation of the formation of irregular secondary (tertiary) dentine.

A **dental base** is a material that is placed on the floor of the cavity preparation in a relatively thick layer. Its purpose is to protect the pulp by providing thermal insulation due to temperature changes and absorbing occlusal forces. It can also be used to line out undercut areas for indirect restorations such as gold or composite inlays.

Cavity varnishes are used to seal the dentinal tubules in order to reduce microleakage that may cause sensitivity, discoloration and bacterial invasion. Dental varnishes are indicated under amalgam restorations and prevent moisture contamination in newly placed glass ionomer restorations. (Cavity varnishes have been largely replaced by dentine bonding agents). However it is not compatible with resin composite materials because it blocks adhesion and has a detrimental effect on the bonding properties. Cavity varnish may be used to protect the external surface of a newly placed glass ionomer cement restoration from early moisture contamination.

Bases and liners are 'sandwiched' between the cavity preparation and the restorative material of the operator's choice; they may be referred to as intermediary materials. Although the function of a base and a liner is pulpal protection, the way this is achieved varies depending on the properties of the materials.

Dental liner	Dental base	Cavity varnish
Glass ionomer	Zinc oxide eugenol	Copal varnish
Calcium hydroxide	Zinc phosphate	
	Glass ionomer	
	Polycarboxylate	
	Flowable resin	

Calcium hydroxide is a dental liner that stimulates the formation of irregular secondary (tertiary) dentine. It also has a function for direct or indirect pulp capping (see Chapter 9), but will only be discussed in this chapter as a *dental liner*.

Material constituents/composition

Most often supplied in a two-paste system – 'catalyst' and 'base'. Constituents vary between manufacturers. The below constituents are specific to Life (Kerr).

Catalyst	Base
Barium sulphate	Calcium hydroxide
Titanium dioxide	Zinc oxide
Methyl salicylate	Butyl benzene sulfonamide

Calcium hydroxide is the active ingredient in the material, and the other ingredients may vary depending on the manufacturer.

Calcium hydroxide may also be supplied in a light-cured form

Light-cured form
Urethane dimethacrylate resin (shrinks on setting)
Calcium hydroxide
Barium sulphate fillers

Properties

- Low thermal conductivity
- Stimulates the production of irregular secondary (tertiary) dentine
- pH of 11–12 (i.e. alkaline)
- Bactericidal properties
- Highly soluble (not applicable to resin version)

Advantages

- Easily manipulated
- Stimulates the formation of irregular secondary (tertiary) dentine

Disadvantages

- Moisture sensitive
- Low strength

LINER AND BASES

Indications and contraindications for use

Indications

- Used in the deepest portion of cavity preparation

- For use with direct or indirect pulp capping

- Only used when within 1–2 mm of pulp or direct pulp capping

- May be used underneath a base

Contraindications

- Cannot be applied thick enough to provide thermal protection for the pulp due to poor strength

Trade names

Trade name	Manufacturer
Dycal® (Figure 7.1a)	Dentsply
Hydrox™ (Figure 7.1b)	Bosworth
Life (Figure 7.1c)	Kerr
VLC Dycal®	Dentsply

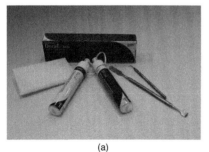
(a)

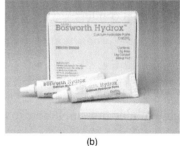
(b)

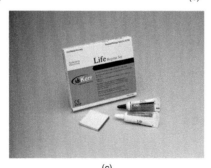
(c)

Figure 7.1 (a) Dycal® – Dentsply. (b) Hydrox™ – Bosworth. (c) Life – Kerr.

Manipulation (Figures 7.2a–7.2c)

Wearing personal protective equipment:

Two-paste system
Step 1

- Dispense equal volumes of both catalyst and base onto a waxed paper pad according to the manufacturer's instructions (use sparingly as not much material is needed)

- Do not allow the two pastes to touch

- Ensure that the correct caps are replaced on the appropriate tube to prevent cross-contamination of the base and catalyst

Step 2

- Mix pastes together in a circular motion until a homogeneous (even) colour is achieved (10–15 seconds)

Step 3

- Pass the material to the operator along with a calcium hydroxide applicator for application

- Have some gauze at hand to wipe the calcium hydroxide instrument in between applications

Step 4

- Receive the calcium hydroxide instrument from the operator

Step 5

- Wipe excess material from the spatula

Step 6

- Dispose of the waxed paper pad and excess material in the contaminated waste bin

Light-cured system
Step 1

- Dispense material

Step 2

- Pass material (usually supplied in syringe form) to the operator

Step 3

- Receive the calcium hydroxide syringe from the operator
- Light cure material as per manufacturer's instructions

Step 4

- Wipe excess material from the calcium hydroxide instrument

Step 5

- Dispose of capsule and/or waxed paper pad in the contaminated waste

Mixing time

- Two-paste system – 10–15 seconds, light cured no mixing

Setting time

- Two-paste system – 1.5–2.5 minutes: light curing material – immediately upon polymerisation

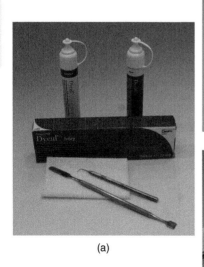
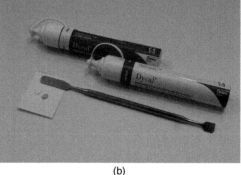
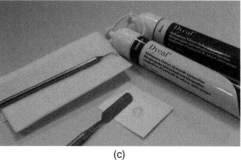

Figure 7.2 (a) Calcium hydroxide set-up. (b) Step 1 – equal volumes of the base and catalyst are dispensed. (c) Step 2 – final mixed material with a homogenous colour achieved.

Instruments and materials used in set-up

- Calcium hydroxide material
- Waxed paper mixing pad
- Mixing spatula
- Calcium hydroxide applicator
- Gauze

Optional:

- Curing light
- Amber light protection shield

CAVITY VARNISH

Cavity varnish is a liquid resin that is used to seal exposed dentinal tubules to reduce sensitivity due to microleakage, to prevent acids from materials entering tubules and to prevent discolouration of the tooth from the metal ions in amalgam. The solvent constituent of the liquid dissolves once the cavity varnish is applied to the tooth surface, which leaves behind a porous layer. Multiple layers may be applied to reach the desired barrier, drying in between applications. Liquid solvent may be added to the cavity varnish to thin it, if it becomes too thick.

Material constituents/composition

Copal resin in a volatile solvent.

Properties

- The solvent constituent evaporates rapidly, leaving the thin insoluble layer sealing the dentinal tubules
- Physical adhesion to tooth structure
- Does not provide thermal insulation
- Non-irritating and non-acidic
- Strong odour and taste
- To be added in very thin layers, allowing to dry in between

LINER AND BASES

Indications and contraindications for use

Indications
- For use under amalgam and to seal the external surface of newly placed glass ionomer restorations

Contraindications
- Contraindicated with the use of resin composites, polymers and glass ionomers (inhibits bonding)

Trade names

Trade name	Manufacturer
Cavity Varnish™ (Figure 7.3a) Copalite	Bosworth (Cooley and Cooley)

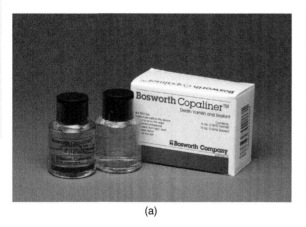 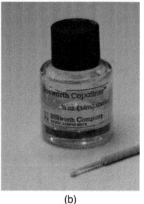

(a)   (b)

Figure 7.3 (a) Cavity varnish™ – Bosworth. (b) Cavity varnish set-up.

Manipulation (Figure 7.3b)

Wearing personal protective equipment:

Step 1

- There is no mixing necessary with cavity varnish
- Remove the cap of the bottle

Step 2

- Using sterile college tweezers and a cotton pellet, or disposable applicator brush (preferred), dip the cotton pellet/disposable applicator into the cavity varnish and dab off the excess

- Replace the cap immediately as cavity varnish evaporates quickly

Step 3

- Pass the college tweezers and cotton pellet/disposable applicator brush to the operator

Step 4

- The operator will dry the surface in between applications using a 3-in-1 syringe/air-water syringe

Step 5

- Using *separate* sterile college tweezers and cotton pellet(s) or new disposable applicator brush(es), repeat step 2 until the desired number of coats has been achieved

Step 6

- Dispose of the cotton pellet(s) and/or disposable applicator brush(es) in the contaminated waste

Instruments and materials used in set-up

- Mouth mirror and handle
- Cavity varnish material
- 2 X college tweezers (locking type preferable)
- Cotton pellets or disposable applicator brushes
- 3-in-1 syringe/air-water syringe

ZINC PHOSPHATE

Zinc phosphate may be used as an insulating base or a luting cement. Zinc phosphate is a material with a moderate solubility as a base and a high solubility

LINER AND BASES

as a luting cement. In this chapter, it will be discussed in the context of a **base** only.

Constituents

Zinc phosphate is supplied in a powder/liquid form and is available in different shades.

Powder (base)	Liquid (acid)
Zinc oxide	Phosphoric acid
Magnesium oxide	Water
	Aluminium and zinc ions

Properties

During manipulation of zinc phosphate, once the powder and liquid are mixed together, heat is produced, i.e. an exothermic reaction takes place. This exothermic reaction speeds up the setting of the material. To control the setting of zinc phosphate, it is always mixed on a *cool*, dry glass slab, and the whole surface area of the slab should be used during the mix to minimize heat production. The manipulation technique is very important as a warm slab, mixing too fast or contamination by water will speed up the setting time of the material. Incorporating the powder increments too fast or too slow will also affect the setting of zinc phosphate. Zinc phosphate is fast setting and has a moderate to high solubility and low acidity (once set). The pH is 1–2 but the acidity decreases over time (about 24 hours).

- Acidic
- Gives off an exothermic reaction (gives out heat when mixed)
- Strong material (reaches two-thirds of strength in less than one hour)
- May be used as a base (thicker mix) or a luting cement (thinner mix)
- Mixing times may be extended by mixing the material over a large surface area (dissipates the heat given off as a result of the exothermic reaction)
- Mixing on a cool glass slab can also extend the working time and allow for greater powder incorporation (gives the material a higher strength and reduces solubility)
- Care must be taken to not reduce the ratio of powder to liquid as this results in a more soluble, more irritant and weaker material

- 50% of the strength of material is reached after 10 minutes, reaching its final strength after 24 hours

Advantages

- Moderate solubility when used as a base and high solubility when used as a luting cement
- Long shelf-life
- Low thermo-conductivity
- Rapid setting time
- Low cost
- Long clinical history

Disadvantages

- Does not release fluoride
- Freshly mixed material has a high acidity (reduces with setting), but has the potential to indirectly cause pulpal irritation (dissolves smear layer)
- Moisture sensitive
- Significant shrinkage during setting
- No adhesive properties
- Brittle

Indications and contraindications for use

Indications
- Used under amalgam restorations as a base providing thermal insulation or as a luting cement
- May be used over a calcium hydroxide liner or cavity varnish (depending on cavity depth)

Contraindications
- Zinc phosphate is acidic at time of placement; therefore, care should be taken to protect the pulp from possible exposure

LINER AND BASES

Trade names

Trade name	Manufacturer
DeTray® (Figure 7.4a)	Dentsply
Flecks® (Figure 7.4b)	Keystone Group
Zinc Cement (Figure 7.4c)	SSWhite
Zinc Phosphate Cement (Figure 7.4d)	Bosworth

LINER AND BASES

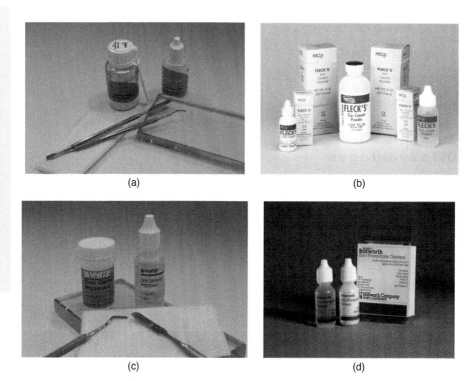

(a)

(b)

(c)

(d)

Figure 7.4 (a) Detray® – Dentsply. (b) Flecks® – Keystone Group. (c) Zinc cement – SSWhite. (d) Zinc phosphate cement – Bosworth.

Manipulation (Figures 7.5a–7.5e)

Zinc phosphate as a base – see Chapter 8 for luting.
   Wearing personal protective equipment:

Step 1

• Ensure that you have a clean, disinfected, cool, dry glass mixing slab

- If cooling the glass slab under cold water, ensure that all moisture is removed prior to dispensing materials (alternatively, place in the fridge until it reaches desired temperature prior to use)

Step 2

- Fluff the zinc phosphate powder in the bottle (shake the bottle, ensuring the lid is securely in place) to disperse powder particles evenly

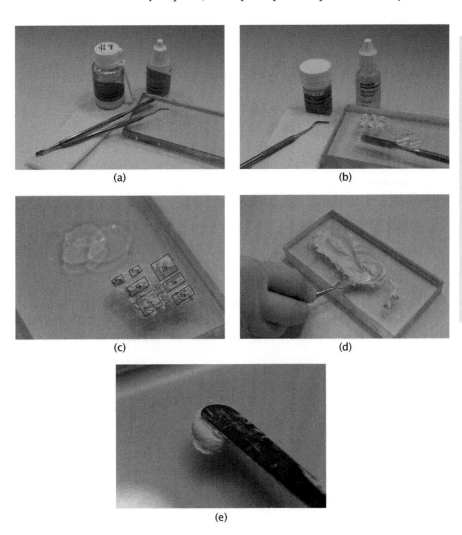

(a)

(b)

(c)

(d)

(e)

Figure 7.5 (a) Zinc phosphate set-up. (b) Step 3 – Zinc phosphate dispensed – powder divided into six equal portions. (c) Step 3 – Zinc phosphate dispensed – powder divided into fractional portions (7.5b and 7.5c are two different techniques for dispensing zinc phosphate powder). (d) Step 5 – figure-of-eight mixing motion. (e) Step 7 – putty-like consistency of zinc phosphate for use as a base.

Step 3

- Dispense the powder on the glass slab according to the manufacturer's instructions, replacing the cap immediately after dispensing (it is
  important that the material is dispensed immediately prior to manipulation – see below). The quantity is determined by the size of the
  restoration

- Manufacturer's instructions vary for the division of powder/liquid ratio, two techniques are shown

Step 4

- Dispense the liquid as per the manufacturer's instructions, according
  to the appropriate amount of powder dispensed (less liquid is used for
  mixing a base consistency than a luting cement)

  *You must take care when mixing zinc phosphate to replace the cap on
  the liquid once it has been dispensed. The material is water based and
  if the cap is left off, the water will evaporate and slow down the setting
  process.*

- To ensure uniform drops, hold the bottle perpendicular to the glass
  slab and immediately replace the cap (see Introductory Chapter)

Step 5

- Mix in the powder increments at 15-second intervals

- Using a Weston spatula (thin, flexible metal spatula) incorporate the first mound of powder into the liquid, spatulating in a
  figure-of-eight motion over the entire surface area of the slab for
  15 seconds

Step 6

- Ensure that all the powder has been incorporated into the liquid and
  then add the second powder increment, following the same mixing
  technique for 15 seconds

Step 7

- Repeat steps 5 and 6 until you have achieved the desired putty-like
  consistency

Step 8

- Using the spatula gather the material in one area and using a plastic
  instrument pass the material to the operator

Step 9

- Have some gauze at hand to wipe away excess cement from the plastic instrument

Step 10

- Immediately clean the spatula and glass slab; if there is not enough time to clean immediately, immerse it in water until cleaning can take place

Mixing time

- 2 minutes

Setting time

- 5–7 minutes

Instruments and materials used in set-up

- Mouth mirror and handle
- Zinc phosphate powder and liquid
- Weston spatula
- Cool, dry glass mixing slab
- Gauze
- Flat plastic

LINER AND BASES

ZINC OXIDE EUGENOL

Zinc oxide eugenol (ZOE) may be used as a base, a temporary restorative material, a temporary luting agent, impression material, bite registration material or a periodontal dressing (different form). In this chapter, it will be discussed in the context of a *base*. ZOE cements are oil-based cements that have a sedative effect on the pulp.

Material constituents/composition

Available in powder and liquid form, two-paste system and capsule form.

Powder (base)	Liquid (acid)
Zinc oxide	Eugenol
White resin	Water
Zinc stearate	Oils
Zinc acetate	

Zinc oxide eugenol is also available in a non-eugenol (does not contain eugenol) form, which is suitable for use in patients having a sensitivity to eugenol. The non-eugenol form contains oils rather than eugenol.

Zinc oxide eugenol is available in two forms. **Type II** is reinforced and contains methyl methacrylate or alumina in the powder and eugenol and ortho-ethoxy benzoic acid in the liquid. These additions reduce the solubility and improve the strength of the material. **Type I** contains none of these additional materials, thereby reducing the strength making it more suitable for temporary restorations.

Properties

- Type I and Type II available
- Type I low strength, Type II (reinforced) moderate strength
- Neutral properties
- Moisture is needed for setting

Advantages

- Antimicrobial
- Good sealing ability

Disadvantages

- Type I has a high solubility and Type II has a moderate to low solubility
- Does not release fluoride
- Type I has a lower strength than Type II, which has moderate strength

Indications and contraindications for use

Indications
- Base

- Temporary filling material

- Luting cement

- Periodontal dressing (different form)

- Temporary cement

- Bite registration material

Contraindications
- Not to be used in conjunction with resin composites as the eugenol contained in zinc oxide eugenol retards the setting

Trade names

Trade name	Manufacturer
B&T®	Dentsply
IRM®	Dentsply
Kalzinol®	Dentsply
Reinforced ZOE Cement (Figure 7.6)	Master-Dent

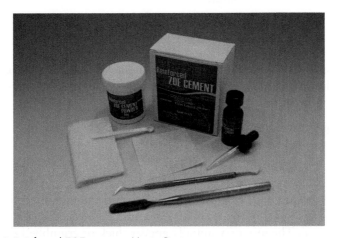

Figure 7.6 Reinforced ZOE cement – Master-Dent.

LINER AND BASES

Manipulation (Figures 7.7a–7.7d)

Wearing personal protective equipment:

Powder/liquid:

Step 1

- Prepare and isolate the tooth appropriately

Step 2

- Dispense the material immediately prior to use

Step 3

- Fluff powder bottle with cap in place (this provides a more consistent volume of powder in each scoop)
- Dispense powder onto waxed paper pad (using measuring scoop, if provided)
- Replace the lid on the powder bottle immediately after dispensing

Step 4

- Divide the zinc oxide eugenol powder into four equal portions using the broad-bladed spatula

Step 5

- Dispense the liquid, holding it perpendicular to the waxed paper pad, following the manufacturer's instructions. A ratio of approximately 3:1 powder to liquid should be used
- Replace the dropper in the bottle

Step 6

- Incorporate the first powder measure into the dispensed liquid. Use the broad part of the spatula to mix in the powder using a 'stropping motion'. The mix may initially appear thick or crumbly; keep mixing with the stropping motion as this will bring out the oil in the mixture, bringing the mix to the desired consistency

Step 7

- Repeat step 6 until the desired consistency is met, which is a putty-like mixture that can be rolled into the shape of a rope or ball for placement using the spatula

Step 8

- Hand the zinc oxide eugenol material to the operator on the waxed paper pad with the operator's choice of hand instrument (usually condenser/plugger or flat plastic instrument)
- Leave a small amount of powder for the operator as it may be used as a separator

Step 9

- Receive the dental instrument from the operator and wipe it clean

Step 10

- Dispose of any waste material and waxed paper pad in the contaminated waste bin

LINER AND BASES

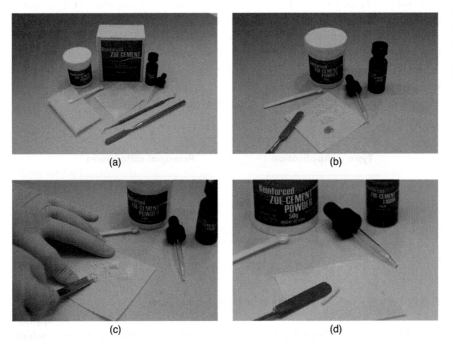

(a)

(b)

(c)

(d)

Figure 7.7 (a) ZOE set-up. (b) Step 4 – ZOE dispensed. (c) Step 6 – 'stropping' mixing motion. (d) Step 7 – putty-like consistency rolled into a rope.

Mixing time

- 30–60 seconds

Setting time

- 7–9 minutes

Instruments and materials used in set-up

- Waxed paper pad
- Broad bladed spatula
- Zinc oxide eugenol powder and liquid, or capsule
- Flat plastic instrument

GLASS IONOMER

Glass ionomers may be used as a restorative material, base, liner or as a luting agent. In this chapter, it will be discussed in the context of a **base**.

Glass ionomers are a diverse group of materials. They are supplied in many different forms. It is the particle size of glass ionomers that dictates their usage. Luting and lining materials have smaller particle sizes than restorative forms of glass ionomer.

Different types of glass Ionomers are listed in the following table:

Type	Application	Principal differences
I	Luting agent	Small particle size
II	Class III and V restorations	Larger particle size
III	Liner or base	Small particle size
IV	Crown and core build-up	Larger particle size

Material constituents/composition

Available in powder/liquid form or pre-measured encapsulated form, which requires titration. May be supplied as conventional or resin-modified glass ionomers.

Powder / liquid:

Powder	Liquid
Aluminosilicate glass • Calcium • Aluminium • Fluoride	Polyacrylic acid Water

Properties

- May be used as luting, lining and restorative (class III and class V in permanent dentition and as a posterior filling material in the primary dentition) materials

- Highest release of fluoride of all restorative materials

- Not as durable as many other materials

- Wear rate is high

- Chemically bonds to enamel, dentine and some metals

- May be used with a conditioner to remove the dentinal smear layer where appropriate

- May be used with calcium hydroxide for pulpal exposures

- Moisture sensitive – both to excessive wetting and excessive drying

Advantages

- Bonds directly to enamel and dentine

- Bonds to base metals

- Does not need to be applied incrementally

- Releases fluoride

- Can be set by polymerisation

Disadvantages

- Aesthetics inferior to composite resin
- Moisture sensitive
- Mixing material is technique sensitive, and the correct liquid / powder ratio must be used (otherwise cement will become weaker with improper mixing proportions); capsulated mixes are preferred for this reason
- Short working time
- Long setting time
- Brittle material
- Needs 24 hours prior to polishing and finishing
- Not as strong as amalgam and composites

Indications and contraindications for use

Indications
- Used for dental liners and bases

Contraindications
- Deep cavity preparations with close proximity to the pulp
- Where it is difficult to achieve good moisture control

Trade names

Trade name	Manufacturer
Riva (self-cure) powder/liquid (Figure 7.8a)	SDI
Riva (self-cure) capsule (Figure 7.8b)	SDI
Vitrebond™ (resin modified) (Figure 7.8c)	3M ESPE

LINER AND BASES

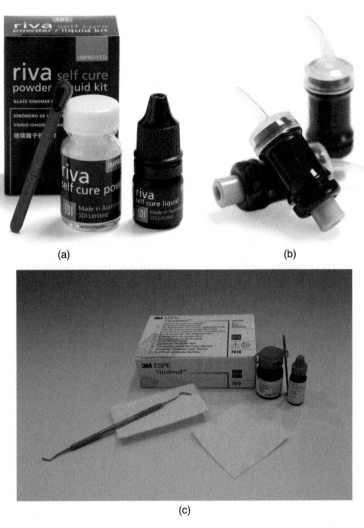

(a)   (b)

(c)

Figure 7.8 (a) Riva self-cure (powder and liquid) – SDI. (b) Riva capsulated form – SDI. (c) Vitrebond™ – 3M ESPS.

Manipulation (Figures 7.9a–7.9c)

Wearing personal protective equipment:

Powder/ liquid form:

Step 1

- Fluff the powder of the glass ionomer by shaking with the lid secured tightly

LINER AND BASES

Step 2

- Using the supplied powder scoop dispense the material as per the manufacturer's instructions
- Dispense the liquid by holding the bottle perpendicular to the waxed paper pad or glass slab to get an accurate drop – replace caps securely
- A waxed paper pad is preferred for mixing for infection control reasons and ease of clean up

Step 3

- Using a Weston spatula (or plastic spatula, if supplied by the manufacturer) divide the powder into two equal portions
- Incorporate the first powder mound into the liquid (following the manufacturer's instructions for timing)

Step 4

- Spatulate the mix over a small surface area using the flat surface of the spatula. Ensure all of the powder is completely incorporated into the liquid before proceeding with the second mound of powder

Step 5

- Incorporate the second mound of powder and mix until a homogenous mix is achieved

Step 6

- Pass the operator a flat plastic instrument with the glass ionomer on the waxed paper pad

Step 7

- Have some gauze ready in case excess cement needs to be wiped away

Step 8

- Dispose of excess cement and the waxed paper pad in the contaminated waste bin
- Ensure the complete removal of cement from the instruments and glass slab (if applicable), as any remaining cement will impede the sterilisation process

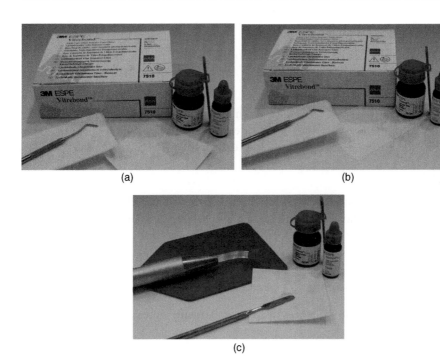

Figure 7.9 (a) Resin-modified glass ionomer set-up. (b) Step 3 – Resin-modified glass ionomer dispensed. (c) Step 5 – Resin-modified glass ionomer mixed.

Mixing time

- 30–60 seconds (follow the manufacturer's instructions)

Working time

- 1.5–2 minutes

Setting time

- Initial setting in the oral cavity is 6–9 minutes from the initiation of the mixture
- Complete setting – several days

Capsule form:

Step 1

- Activate the glass ionomer capsule (following the manufacturer's instructions)

Step 2

- Avoiding cross-contamination of the amalgamator, load the activated glass ionomer capsule into the amalgamator. It is easiest to load one end of the capsule first
- Close the cover of the amalgamator over the glass ionomer capsule. This cover is in place for the safety of the operator in the event that the glass ionomer capsule becomes displaced from the amalgamator

Step 3

- Select the time for the glass ionomer to be titrated by the dial or the button (follow the manufacturer's instructions when selecting titration time)

Step 4

- Push the button to activate the trituration of the glass ionomer
- The amalgamator will stop automatically once the time has been reached

Step 5

- Remove the glass ionomer capsule from the amalgamator and load it into the applicator/gun

Step 6

- Pass the applicator/gun to the operator handle first

Step 7

- Have some gauze ready, if excess cement needs to be wiped away

Step 8

- Dispose of excess cement and the waxed paper pad in the contaminated waste bin
- Ensure the complete removal of cement from the instruments as any remaining cement will impede the sterilisation process

Instruments and materials used in set-up

Common to both powder/liquid form and capsule form:

- Instrument set-up

- Gauze
- Flat plastic instrument

Powder/liquid form:

- Glass ionomer powder and liquid
- Weston spatula
- Waxed paper pad or glass slab

Capsule form:

- Glass ionomer capsule
- Amalgamator

POLYCARBOXYLATE CEMENTS (ZINC POLYCARBOXYLATE CEMENTS)

Polycarboxylate cement is a derivative of zinc phosphate cement in which the zinc phosphate has been replaced with a polyacrylic acid. It has the ability to bond to both enamel and dentine.

Material constituents/composition

Supplied in powder and liquid forms:

Powder	Liquid
Zinc oxide	Polyacrylic acid
Magnesium oxide	Water

Properties

- Acceptable to mix on either a waxed paper pad or glass slab
- Mixing polycarboxylate cement on a cool glass slab enables extension of the working time

- Reaches 80% of its final setting in one hour
- Do not store the liquid in the fridge as this will cause it to gel

Advantages

- Does not release fluoride, although some materials have added properties which allow fluoride release
- Bonds to enamel, dentine and alloys
- Low irritation
- Easy manipulation

Disadvantages

- Short mixing/working times
- Sensitive to manipulation techniques
- Lower compressive strength when compared to zinc phosphate

Indications and contraindications for use

Indications
- Base material
- Cementation of metal crowns and bridges (also suitable for porcelain fused to metal crowns and bridges) – luting consistency
- Orthodontic bands and appliances – luting consistency

Contraindications
- Does not bond well to untreated gold restorations

Trade names

Trade name	Manufacturer
Poly F Plus® (Figure 7.10)	Dentsply

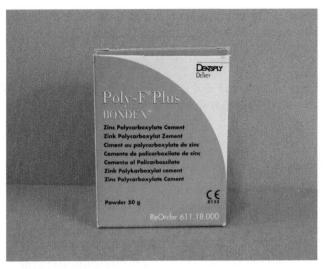

Figure 7.10 Poly-F® Plus – Dentsply.

Manipulation (Figures 7.11a–7.11c)

Wearing personal protective equipment:

Step 1

- Ensure you have a clean, disinfected, cool, dry glass mixing slab or waxed paper pad (operator preference)
- If the chosen method to cool the glass slab is under cold water, ensure that all moisture is removed prior to dispensing materials

Step 2

- Fluff the polycarboxylate powder in the bottle (shake the bottle, ensuring the lid is securely in place)

Step 3

- Dispense the powder on the glass slab or waxed paper pad according to the manufacturer's instructions, replacing the cap immediately after dispensing (use dispensing scoop, if provided)
- Dispense liquid as per the manufacturer's instructions, according to the appropriate amount of powder dispensed (most often one scoop to two drops of water – luting, and two scoops to two drops of water base consistency)

- To ensure uniform drops of the liquid, hold the bottle vertically during dispensing and immediately replace the cap

Step 4

- Spatulate the powder and liquid together quickly using a folding motion for 15–20 seconds using a Weston spatula

Step 5

- The material will appear glossy once mixed
- Mix to a putty consistency

Step 6

- Using the spatula gather the material into one area and extend the material and flat plastic (or the desired instrument) to the operator

Step 7

- Have some gauze at hand to wipe away excess cement from the plastic instrument

Step 8

- Immediately clean the spatula and glass slab. If there is not enough time to clean immediately, immerse them in water until cleaning can take place. Dispose of gauze and waxed paper in the contaminated waste bin

Mixing time

- 15–20 seconds

Setting time

- 6–9 minutes

Working time

- 2.5–3.5 minutes

Instruments and materials used in set-up

- Polycarboxylate powder and liquid
- Weston spatula

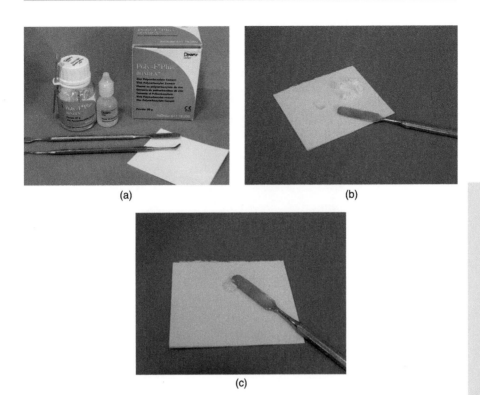

(a) (b)

(c)

Figure 7.11 (a) Polycarboxylate cement set-up. (b) Step 3 – Polycarboxylate cement dispensed. (c) Step 6 – Final desired putty consistency of polycarboxylate cement.

- Cool, dry glass slab or waxed paper pad – operator's preference
- Gauze

Flowable composites may also be used as dental liners (see Chapter 5).

FURTHER READING

Craig, R.G., Powers, J.M. and Wataha, J.C. (2004). *Dental Materials: Properties and Manipulation*. 8th edn. Philadelphia: Mosby.

Hilton TJ. (1996). Cavity sealers, liners, and bases: Current philosophies and indications for use. *Operative Dentistry*, **21**, 134–146.

Kerr, C.A. (2006). *Life Catalyst Paste Material Safety Data Sheet*. Available online at http://www.kerrtotalcare.com/msds/kerrdental/us/english/LifeCatalystPaste.pdf. (Accessed: 12 March 2009).

Kerr, CA. (2006) *Life Base Paste Material Safety Data Sheet*. Available online at http://www.kerrtotalcare.com/msds/kerrdental/us/english/LifeCatalystPaste.pdf. (Accessed: 12 March 2009).

LINER AND BASES

Chapter 8
Dental cements

DEFINITION

A luting cement is a material that bonds, seals or cements objects together (Figure 8.1a–c). It should have low solubility, low viscosity and high fracture resistance. Luting cements are used in dentistry in order to cement crowns, bridges and appliances (e.g. orthodontic appliances) either temporarily or permanently. Depending on the needs of the treatment, the operator will choose the cement based on strength, antibacterial properties, ability to create a good marginal seal, ability to be used with an adhesive, solubility, tensile strength, resistance to wear, ease of manipulation, translucency and operator's preference. There is not one luting agent that will meet the desired needs in all situations, hence the reason for a large number of products available for this use.

ZINC PHOSPHATE

Although zinc phosphate has a function as a base (see Chapter 7), it may also be used as a *luting* cement. It will be discussed in this context in this chapter.

Material constituents/composition

Powder	Liquid
Zinc oxide	Phosphoric acid
Magnesium oxide	Water
	Aluminium and zinc ions

Properties

Once the powder and liquid are mixed together, heat is produced, i.e. an exothermic reaction takes place. This reaction speeds up the setting of the material. To control the setting of zinc phosphate, it should always be mixed on a *cool*, dry glass slab, and the whole surface area of the slab should be used during the mix to minimise heat production. The manipulation technique is very important, as a warm slab, mixing too fast, or contamination by water may speed up the setting time of the material. Incorporating the powder increments too fast or too slow will also affect the setting of zinc phosphate. Zinc phosphate

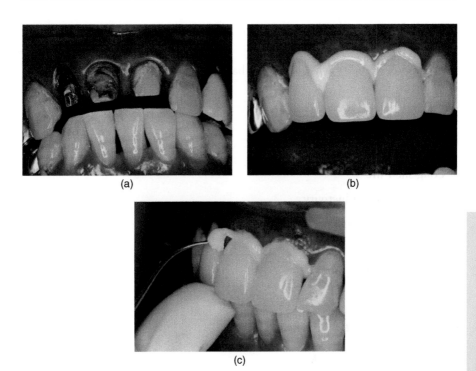

(a)

(b)

(c)

Figure 8.1 (a) Teeth prepared for crowns. (b) Crowns cemented in place with a luting cement. (c) Operator holding the crowns in place until the initial set of the desired luting cement. (Photos courtesy of Dr. Shuichitsubura).

is fast setting and has a moderate to high solubility and low acidity (once set). The pH is 1–2 but the acidity decreases over time (about 24 hours).

- Acidic
- Gives off an exothermic reaction (gives out heat when mixed)
- Strong material (reaches two-thirds of strength in less than one hour)
- May be used as a base (thicker mix) or a luting cement (thinner mix)
- Mixing times may be extended by mixing the material over a large surface area (dissipates the heat given off as a result of the exothermic reaction)
- Mixing on a cool glass slab can also extend the working time and allow for greater powder incorporation (gives the material a higher strength and reduces solubility)
- Care must be taken to not reduce the ratio of powder to liquid as this results in a more soluble, more irritant and weaker material

DENTAL CEMENTS

- 50% of the strength of the material is reached after 10 minutes, reaching its final strength after 24 hours

- Moderate solubility when used as a base and high solubility when used as a luting cement

Advantages

- Long shelf-life

- Low thermo-conductivity

- Rapid setting time

- Low cost

- Long clinical history

Disadvantages

- Does not release fluoride

- Freshly mixed material has a high acidity (reduces with setting), but has the potential to cause pulpal irritation

- Moisture sensitive

- Slight shrinkage during setting

- No adhesive properties

- Brittle

Indications and contraindications for use

Indications
- Permanent cementation of crowns, bridges, inlays, onlays, orthodontic appliances and orthodontic bands

Contraindications
- Zinc phosphate is acidic at the time of placement, and care should be taken to protect the pulp

Trade names

Trade name	Manufacturer
DeTray® (Figure 8.2a)	Dentsply
Flecks® (Figure 8.2b)	Keystone Group
Zinc Cement (Figure 8.2c)	SSWhite
Zinc Phosphate Cement (Figure 8.2d)	Bosworth

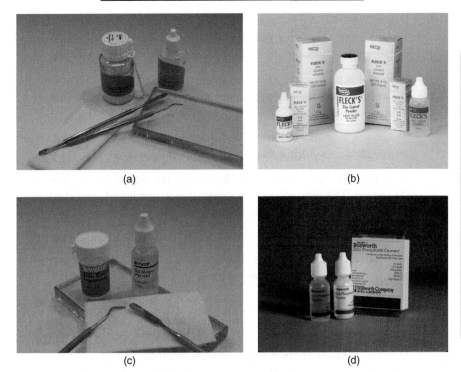

(a)　　　　　　　　　　(b)

(c)　　　　　　　　　　(d)

DENTAL CEMENTS

Figure 8.2 (a) DeTray® – Dentsply. (b) Flecks® – Keystone group. (c) Zinc Cement – SS White. (d) Zinc Phosphate Cement – Bosworth.

Manipulation (Figures 8.3a–8.3e)

This is the same manipulation technique as mixing zinc phosphate as a base, except with altered powder/liquid ratios, mixing times and final consistency. Wearing personal protective equipment:

Step 1

- Tooth is appropriately prepared and isolated

- Ensure you have a clean, disinfected, cool, dry glass mixing slab
- If the chosen method is to cool the glass slab under cold water, ensure that all moisture is removed prior to dispensing materials

Step 2

- Fluff the zinc phosphate powder in the bottle (shake the bottle, ensuring the lid is securely in place)

Step 3

- Dispense the powder on the glass slab according to the manufacturer's instructions, replacing the cap immediately after dispensing
- Dispense liquid as per the manufacturer's instructions, according to the appropriate amount of powder dispensed (more liquid is added for a luting consistency than a base)
- To ensure uniform drops of the liquid, hold the bottle perpendicular to the glass slab during dispensing and immediately replace the cap
- Care must be taken to replace the cap on the liquid once it has been dispensed. The zinc phosphate material is water based, and the water will evaporate if the cap is left off, which will prolong the setting time

Step 4

- Section powder into increments according to the manufacturer's instructions (two techniques are shown)

Step 5

- Mix in powder increments at 15-second intervals
- Using a Weston spatula (thin, flexible spatula) incorporate the first mound of powder into the liquid, spatulating in a figure-of-eight motion over the entire surface area of the slab for 15 seconds

Step 6

- Ensure that all the powder has been incorporated into the liquid and add the second powder increment, following the same mixing technique for 15 seconds

Step 7

- Repeat steps 5 and 6 until you have achieved the desired creamy consistency (the mixed material should form a 'string' from the spatula to the glass slab when the spatula is lifted approximately an inch (2 cm) above the glass slab)

DENTAL CEMENTS

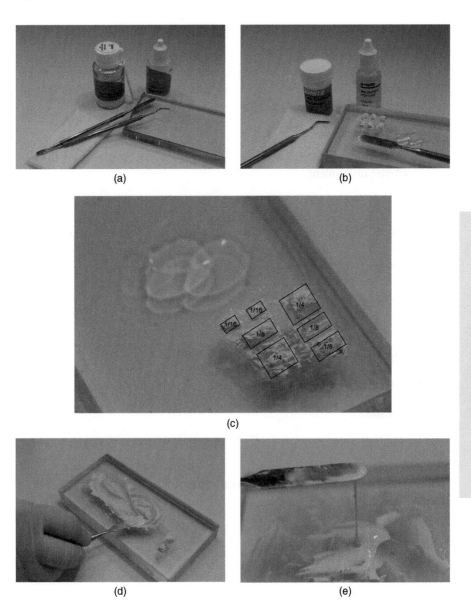

Figure 8.3 (a) Zinc phosphate set-up. (b) Step 4 – Zinc phosphate dispensed – powder divided into six equal portions. (c) Step 4 – Zinc phosphate dispensed – powder divided into fractional portions (8.3b and 8.3c are two different techniques for dispensing zinc phosphate powder). (d) Step 5 – figure-of-eight mixing motion. (e) Step 7 – luting consistency of zinc phosphate (2cm 'string' from glass slab to spatula).

DENTAL CEMENTS

Step 8

- Using the spatula, gather the material into one area and use a flat plastic instrument to load the restoration or prosthesis to be cemented under the direction of the operator, alternatively pass the material and the flat plastic instrument to the operator for loading

Step 9

- Have some gauze at hand to wipe away excess cement from the flat plastic instrument

Step 10

- Immediately clean the spatula and glass slab; if there is not enough time to clean immediately, immerse the slab and spatula in water until cleaning can take place

Mixing time

- 60–90 seconds

Working time

- 3–6 minutes

Setting time

- 5–14 minutes

Instruments and materials used in set-up

- Zinc phosphate powder and liquid
- Weston spatula
- Cool, dry glass slab
- Gauze
- Flat plastic instrument

POLYCARBOXYLATE CEMENTS (ZINC POLYCARBOXYLATE CEMENTS)

Polycarboxylate cement is a derivative of zinc phosphate cement in which the zinc phosphate has been replaced with a polyacrylic acid. It has the ability to bond to both enamel and dentine.

Material constituents/composition

Supplied in powder and liquid forms:

Powder	Liquid
Zinc oxide	Polyacrylic acid
Magnesium oxide	Water

Properties

- Acceptable to mix polycarboxylate cement on either a waxed paper pad or a glass slab
- Mixing polycarboxylate cement on a cooled glass slab enables extension of the working time
- Reaches 80% of its final setting in one hour
- Do not store the liquid in the fridge as this will cause it to gel

Advantages

- Does not release fluoride, although some materials have added properties which allow fluoride release
- Bonds to enamel, dentine and alloys
- Low irritation
- Easy manipulation

Disadvantages

- Short mixing/working times
- Sensitive to manipulation techniques
- Lower compressive strength when compared to zinc phosphate

Indications and contraindications for use

Indications
- Cementation of metal crowns and bridges (also suitable for porcelain fused to metal crowns and bridges)
- Orthodontic bands and appliances

Contraindications

- Does not bond well to untreated gold restorations

Trade names

Trade name	Manufacturer
Poly-F® Plus (Figure 8.4) (this material has added properties to release fluoride)	Dentsply

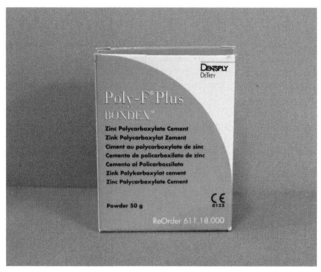

Figure 8.4 Poly-F® Plus – Dentsply.

Manipulation (Figures 8.5a–8.5c)

Wearing personal protective equipment:

Step 1

- Ensure you have a clean, disinfected, cool, dry glass mixing slab or waxed paper pad (operator preference)
- If the chosen method to cool the glass slab is under cold water, ensure that all moisture is removed prior to dispensing materials

Step 2

- Fluff the polycarboxylate powder in the bottle (shake the bottle, ensuring the lid is securely in place)

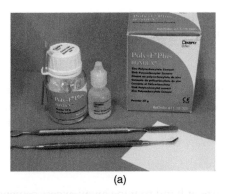

(a)

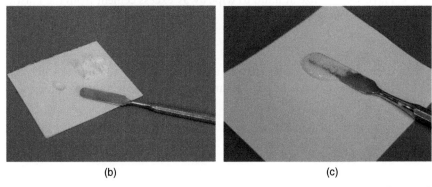

(b)   (c)

Figure 8.5 (a) Polycarboxylate cement set-up. (b) Step 3 – Polycarboxylate cement dispensed. (c) Step 6 – Final desired luting consistency of polycarboxylate cement.

Step 3

- Dispense the powder on the glass slab according to the manufacturer's instructions, replacing the cap immediately after dispensing (use dispensing scoop, if provided)

- Dispense liquid as per the manufacturer's instructions, according to the appropriate amount of powder dispensed

- To ensure uniform drops of the liquid, hold the bottle perpendicular to the mixing surface during dispensing and immediately replace the cap

Step 4

- Spatulate the powder and liquid together quickly using a folding motion for 30–60 seconds using a Weston spatula

Step 5

- The material will appear glossy once mixed and should stick to the spatula and glass slab when suspending the spatula above the glass

DENTAL CEMENTS

slab (if the gloss disappears from the material, do not use it as this indicates initial setting has commenced)

Step 6

- Using the spatula, gather the material into one area and using a flat plastic instrument apply to the prosthesis or restoration to be cemented or pass the material and the flat plastic to the operator to apply (operator's preference)

Step 7

- Have some gauze at hand to wipe away excess cement from the plastic instrument

Step 8

- Immediately clean the spatula and glass slab; if there is not enough time to clean immediately, immerse them in water until cleaning can take place

Mixing time

- 30–40 seconds

Setting time

- 6–9 minutes

Working time

- 2.5–3.5 minutes

Instruments and materials used in set-up

- Polycarboxylate powder and liquid
- Weston spatula
- Cool, dry glass slab or waxed paper pad – operator's preference
- Gauze
- Flat plastic instrument

GLASS IONOMER

Glass ionomer may be used as a restorative material, base, liner or as a luting agent. Glass ionomer luting cements differ from restorative materials by having a smaller particle size. In this chapter, they will be discussed in the context of a **luting cement**.

Glass ionomers, which are a diverse group of materials, are supplied in many different forms. It is the particle size of glass ionomers that dictates their usage. Luting and lining materials have smaller particle sizes than restorative forms of glass ionomer.

Glass ionomers:

Type	Application	Principal differences
I	Luting agent	Small particle size
II	Class III and V restorations	Larger particle size
III	Liner or base	Small particle size
IV	Crown and core build-up	Larger particle size

Material constituents/composition

Glass ionomers are available in powder and liquid forms or pre-measured encapsulated forms that require titration. They may be supplied as conventional or resin-modified glass ionomers.

Powder /liquid:

Powder	Liquid
Aluminosilicate glass	Polyacrylic acid
• Calcium	Water
• Aluminium	
• Fluoride	

Properties

- May be used as luting, lining and restorative materials (class III and class V in permanent dentition and as a posterior filling material in the primary dentition)

- Highest release of fluoride of all restorative materials

- Not as durable as many other materials

- Wear rate is high

- Chemically bonds to enamel, dentine and some metals

DENTAL CEMENTS

- May be used with a conditioner to remove the dentinal smear layer where appropriate
- May be used with calcium hydroxide for pulpal exposures
- Moisture sensitive – both to excessive wetting and excessive drying

Advantages

- Bonds directly to enamel and dentine
- Bonds to base metals
- Does not need to be applied incrementally
- Fluoride release
- Can be set by polymerisation

Disadvantages

- Aesthetics inferior to composite resin
- Moisture sensitive
- Mixing material is technique sensitive and the correct liquid/powder ratio must be used (otherwise the cement will become weaker with improper mixing proportions); capsulated mixes are preferred for this reason
- Short working time
- Long setting time
- Brittle material
- Translucency of glass ionomer is not as good as composite
- Needs 24 hours prior to polishing and finishing
- Not as strong as amalgam and composites

Indications and contraindications for use

Indications
- Used for permanent cementation of crowns and bridges

Contraindications
- Suggested to use a calcium hydroxide liner under glass ionomer restorative materials if preparation is close to the pulp

DENTAL CEMENTS

Trade names

Trade name	Manufacturer
AquaCem®	Dentsply
Fuji I	GC America
Ketac™ Cem powder/liquid form (Figure 8.6a)	3M ESPE
Ketac™ Cem capsule form (Figure 8.6b)	3M ESPE
RelyX™ Unicem	3M ESPE
Riva Luting powder/liquid form (Figure 8.6c)	SDI
Riva Luting capsule form (Figure 8.6d)	SDI

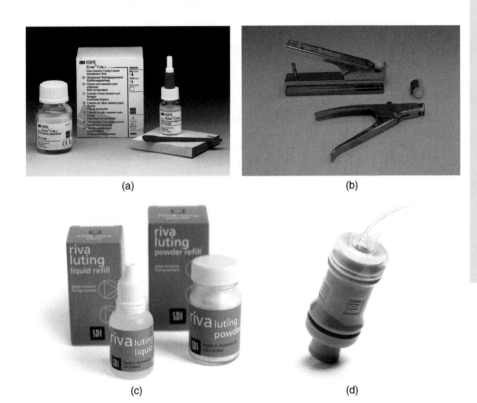

(a)　　　　　　　　　　　　　　(b)

(c)　　　　　　　　　　　　　　(d)

Figure 8.6 (a) Ketac™ Cem powder/liquid form – 3M ESPE. (b) Ketac™ Cem capsule form – 3M ESPE. (c) Riva luting powder/liquid – SDI. (d) Riva luting capsule form – SDI.

DENTAL CEMENTS

Manipulation (Figures 8.7a–8.7c)

Wearing personal protective equipment:

Powder/liquid form:

Step 1

- Fluff the powder of the glass ionomer by shaking with the lid secured tightly

Step 2

- Using the supplied powder scoop dispense the material as per the manufacturer's instructions
- Dispense the liquid by holding the bottle perpendicular to the mixing surface (a waxed paper pad or glass slab) to get an accurate drop – replace caps securely
- A waxed paper pad is preferred for mixing for infection control reasons and ease of clean-up

Step 3

- Using a Weston spatula divide the powder into two equal portions
- Incorporate the first powder mound into the liquid (following the manufacturer's instructions for timing)

Step 4

- Spatulate the mix over a small surface area using the flat surface of the spatula. Ensure all of the powder is completely incorporated into the liquid before proceeding to the second mound of powder

Step 5

- Incorporate the second mound of powder and mix until a homogenous mix is achieved

Step 6

- Pass the operator a flat plastic instrument with the glass ionomer on the waxed paper pad, alternatively the dental nurse may add the cement to the restoration to be cemented prior to handing to the operator
- If you are adding the cement to the restoration, ensure you hand it to the operator so that they can pick it up and efficiently place it in the mouth (i.e. if the restoration is a crown, once the cement is added, extend the crown in the palm of your hand, with the crown occlusal/incisal edge facing up)

DENTAL CEMENTS

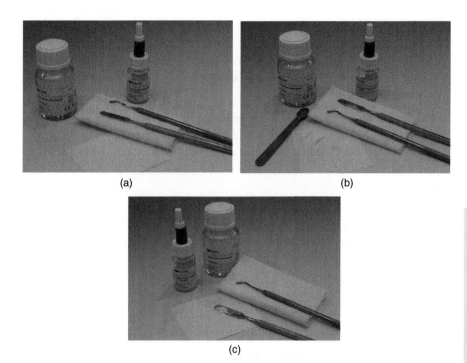

Figure 8.7 (a) Glass ionomer set up. (b) Step 3 – glass ionomer luting cement dispensed. (c) Step 5 – glass ionomer luting cement final homogenous mix.

Step 7

- Have some gauze ready if there is excess cement that needs to be wiped away

Step 8

- Dispose of excess cement and the waxed paper pad in the contaminated waste bin
- Ensure the complete removal of cement from the instruments and glass slab (if applicable) as any remaining cement will impede the sterilisation process

Capsule form:

Step 1

- Activate the glass ionomer capsule (following the manufacturer's instructions)

Step 2

- Avoiding cross-contamination of the amalgamator, load the activated glass ionomer capsule into the amalgamator. It is easiest to load one end of the capsule first
- Close the cover of the amalgamator over the glass ionomer capsule. This cover is in place for the safety of the operator in the event that the glass ionomer capsule becomes displaced from the amalgamator

Step 3

- Select the time for the glass ionomer to be titrated by the dial or the button (follow the manufacturer's instructions when selecting titration time)

Step 4

- Push the button to activate the trituration of the glass ionomer
- The amalgamator will stop automatically once the time has been reached

Step 5

- Remove the glass ionomer capsule from the amalgamator and load it into the applicator/gun

Step 6

- Pass the applicator/gun to the operator handle first

Step 7

- Have some gauze ready if excess cement needs to be wiped away

Step 8

- Dispose of excess cement and the waxed paper pad in the contaminated waste bin
- Ensure the complete removal of cement from the instruments as any remaining cement will impede the sterilisation process

Mixing time

- 30–60 seconds (follow the manufacturer's instructions)

Working time

- 1.5–2 minutes

Setting time

- Initial setting in the oral cavity is 6–9 minutes from the initiation of the mixture
- Complete setting – several days

Instruments and materials used in set-up

Common to both powder/liquid form and capsule form:

- Gauze
- Flat plastic instrument

Powder/liquid form:

- Glass ionomer powder and liquid
- Weston spatula
- Waxed paper pad or glass slab

Capsule form:

- Glass ionomer capsule
- Amalgamator
- Glass ionomer gun/dispenser

ZINC OXIDE EUGENOL

Zinc oxide eugenol (ZOE) may be used as a base, a temporary restorative material, a temporary luting agent, a bite registration or as a periodontal dressing (in a different formulation). In this chapter, it will be discussed in

DENTAL CEMENTS

the context of a *luting material and temporary cement.* ZOE cements are oil-based cements that have a sedative effect on the pulp.

Due to the sedative effect on the pulp, ZOE is particularly useful for luting where there is exposed dentine. The temporary cement form of ZOE is useful for short-term cementation of temporary or permanent crowns. It is available in a two-paste system containing either eugenol or a system with no eugenol.

Material constituents/composition

It is available in powder, liquid or capsule form or as a two-paste system.

Powder (base)	Liquid (acid)
Zinc oxide	Eugenol
Rosin	Water
Zinc stearate	Oils
Zinc acetate	

Zinc oxide eugenol is available in two forms. **Type II** – reinforced, contains methyl methacrylate or alumina in the powder and eugenol and ortho-ethoxy benzoic acid in the liquid. These additions reduce the solubility and improve the strength of the material. **Type I** contains none of these additional materials, thereby reducing the strength and making it more suitable for temporary situations.

The non-eugenol (not containing eugenol) is suitable for use in patients having sensitivity to eugenol and/or when adhesive bonding is anticipated. The non-eugenol form contains oils rather than eugenol.

Properties

- Type I and Type II available

- Type I low strength, Type II (reinforced) moderate strength

- Neutral properties

- Moisture is needed for setting

Advantages

- Antimicrobial

- Good sealing ability

DENTAL CEMENTS

Disadvantages

- Type I has a high solubility and Type II has a moderate to low solubility
- Does not release fluoride
- Type I has a lower strength than Type II, which has moderate strength

Indications and contraindications for use

Indications
- Base
- Temporary filling material
- Luting cement
- Periodontal dressing
- Temporary cement
- Bite registration material

Contraindications
- Should not be used in conjunction with resin composites as the eugenol contained in zinc oxide eugenol retards the setting

Trade names

Trade name	Manufacturer
NexTemp™ (non-eugenol)	Premier
Nogenol™ (non-eugenol)	GC America
Temp-Bond Clear (Figure 8.8a)	Kerr
Temp-Bond Unidose Packs (Figure 8.8b)	Kerr
Temp-Bond (Figure 8.8c)	Kerr
Temp-Bond NE (non-eugenol) (Figure 8.8d)	Kerr

DENTAL CEMENTS

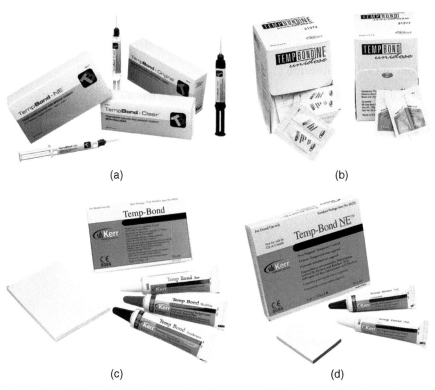

(a)   (b)

(c)   (d)

Figure 8.8 (a) Temp-Bond clear, original and non-eugenol. (b) Temp-Bond unidose packs.
(c) Temp-Bond original. (d) Temp-Bond NE.

Manipulation (Figures 8.9a–8.9c)

Wearing personal protective equipment:
Two-paste-system-temporary cement (non-eugenol and eugenol type):

Step 1

- Prepare and isolate the tooth appropriately

Step 2

- Dispense the material immediately prior to use

Step 3

- Dispense equal lengths of base and catalyst onto a paper mixing pad
- Ensure that the two pastes do not contact each other

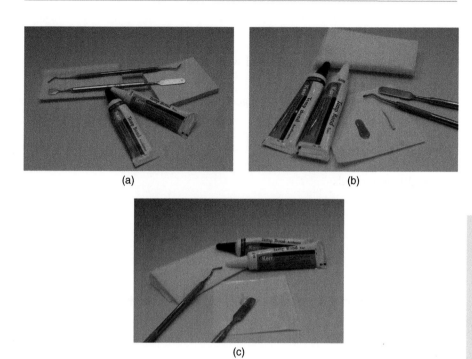

Figure 8.9 (a) Zinc oxide eugenol temporary cement set up. (b) Step 3 – Zinc oxide eugenol temporary cement dispensed. (c) Step 5 – Zinc oxide eugenol temporary cement homogeneous mix.

Step 4

- Using a Weston spatula incorporate the two pastes together using a swirling motion and mix until a homogenous mix is achieved
- The resulting mix should appear to be creamy and uniform in colour

Step 5

- Using the edge of the Weston spatula gather the material into the middle of the waxed paper pad

Step 6

- Using a flat plastic instrument to load the material into the prosthesis, or alternately extend the mixed material and flat plastic to the operator to load

Step 7

- Receive the dental instrument from the operator and wipe it clean

Step 8

- Dispose of waste material and waxed paper pad in the contaminated waste bin

(NB: Manipulation is the same for eugenol and non-eugenol containing temporary cements.)

Mixing time

- 20–30 seconds

Setting time

- 2–4 minutes

Instruments and materials used in set-up

- Waxed paper pad
- Weston spatula
- Zinc oxide eugenol material
- Flat plastic hand instrument
- Gauze

RESIN CEMENTS

Resin cements are available in light cure, dual cure and chemical cure forms. They bond to enamel and dentine and are used for permanent cementation of endodontic posts, orthodontic brackets, porcelain and metal crowns and bridges, porcelain and metal inlays and onlays and veneers. Resin cements are extremely varied, and for this reason they will not be highlighted individually and the information provided in this text is generic. Consult the manufacturer's instructions for indications, contraindications, constituents and manipulation instructions.

Material constituents/composition

Constituents of resin cements are variable depending on the product and manufacturer. Consult the manufacturer for constituents of individual products.

DENTAL CEMENTS

Properties

- Prosthesis may require sandblasting prior to placement to improve retention
- Alloys and ceramics may need to be etched and treated with a coupling agent prior to using a resin cement (a coupling agent is used to create a bond with the resin cement)
- Shade selection available

Advantages

- Aesthetic

Disadvantages

- Increased chairside time needed when using resin cements as they require complex manipulation
- Extremely technique sensitive
- Expensive

Indications and contraindications for use

Indications
- Permanent cementation of inlays, onlays, crowns, bridges, veneers, orthodontic brackets and endodontic posts

Contraindications
- Unsuitable for use in situations where there may be difficulty to maintain good moisture control

Trade names

Trade name	Manufacturer
Calibra	Dentsply
IntegraCem™ (Figure 8.10a)	Premier Dental
Nexus® (Figure 8.10b)	Kerr
Panavia F (8.10c)	Kuraray America
RelyX™ Unicem	3M ESPE
Variolink II	Ivoclar Vivadent

DENTAL CEMENTS

DENTAL CEMENTS

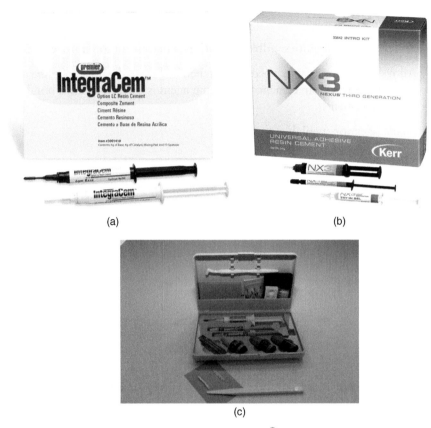

(a)   (b)

(c)

Figure 8.10 (a) IntegraCem™ – Premier Dental. (b) Nexus® 3 – Kerr. (c) Panavia F Light – Kuraray America.

Manipulation

Refer to individual materials manufacturer's instructions; these products are too varied to present generic manipulation instructions.

Instruments and materials used in set-up

- Waxed paper pad
- Plastic mixing spatula (usually supplied with the kit)
- Material – syringe or two-paste system
- Primers, bonding agents and etch as indicated by procedure

- Disposable brushes for applying primers, bonding agents and etch (see the note below)

- Dispensing well for bonding agent, with amber shield to protect from light

- Amber light protection shield

- Curing light

- Flat plastic hand instrument

- Gauze

NB: Due to the complexity of using resin cements, it is important for the dental nurse to use colour-coded, single-use applicator brushes for easy recognition by both the dental nurse and the operator and to avoid cross-contamination of products.

FURTHER READING

Burke, F.J.T. (2005). Trends in indirect dentistry: 3. Luting materials. *Dental Update* **32**: 251–260.

DENTAL CEMENTS

Chapter 9
Endodontic materials

Endodontics is the specialty of dentistry that focuses on the management of prevention, diagnosis and treatment of diseases of the dental pulp and peri-radicular tissues (region around the root of the tooth).

Dental materials have an important role within endodontics. Along with specialised hand and finger instruments, they facilitate capping exposed pulp, cleaning and shaping the root canal, obturating of the root canal and providing a seal after obturation to prevent contamination of the root canal.

Rubber dam should be routinely used during endodontic treatment to provide the most effective moisture control, safety and cross-infection control.

PULP CAPPING

Pulp capping is a procedure that aims to protect the dental pulp and allows for self-repair of the pulpal exposure. Pulpal exposure occurs most often as a result of trauma, tooth wear, dental caries or accidental exposure during a restorative procedure. Direct pulp capping refers to the procedure of placing a dental material (most often calcium hydroxide) directly over the exposed (or nearly exposed) dental pulp to stimulate reparative or irregular secondary (tertiary) dentine. Indirect pulp capping is the procedure of leaving a thin layer of demineralised dentine over the pulp and placing a dental material (most often calcium hydroxide) over this layer. Removing the source of infection, leaving a small amount of demineralised uninfected dentine and adding calcium hydroxide can encourage the re-mineralisation of the remaining dentine and avoid the risk of pulpal exposure by removing the thin layer of demineralised dentine. Calcium hydroxide is used for pulp capping because of its antibacterial properties and its ability to stimulate the formation of irregular secondary (tertiary) dentine. Mineral Trioxide Aggregate is also indicated for this use (see p. 145).

CALCIUM HYDROXIDE

Calcium hydroxide is a dental liner (see Chapter 7) that stimulates the formation of irregular secondary (tertiary) dentine. It will be discussed in this chapter as a *pulp capping material*.

Material constituents/composition

Most often supplied in a two-paste system – 'catalyst' and 'base'. Constituents vary between manufacturers. The constituents listed below are specific to Life (Kerr, 2006).

Catalyst	Base
Barium sulphate	Calcium hydroxide
Titanium dioxide	Zinc oxide
Methyl salicylate	Butyl benzene solfonamide

Calcium hydroxide is the active ingredient in the material, and the other ingredients may vary depending on the manufacturer.

Calcium hydroxide may also be supplied in a light-cured form:

Light-cured form
Urethane dimethacrylate resin
Calcium hydroxide
Barium sulphate fillers

Properties

- Low thermal conductivity
- Stimulates the production of irregular secondary (tertiary) dentine
- pH of 11–12 (i.e. alkaline)
- Bactericidal
- Highly soluble (with the exception of the visible light-cured form)

Advantages

- Easily manipulated
- Stimulates the formation of irregular secondary (tertiary) dentine

Disadvantages

- Moisture sensitive
- Low strength
- Opaque
- Very soluble

ENDODONTIC MATERIALS

Indications and contraindications for use

Indications
- For use with direct or indirect pulp capping within 2 mm of pulp
- For use under permanent restorative materials
- Used in the deepest portion of cavity preparation
- May be used underneath a base

Contraindications
- Cannot be applied in a thick layer

Trade names

Trade name	Manufacturer
Dycal® (Figure 9.1a)	Dentsply
Hydrox™ (Figure 9.1b)	Bosworth
Life (Figure 9.1c)	Kerr
VLC Dycal®	Dentsply

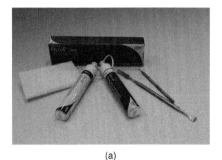
(a)

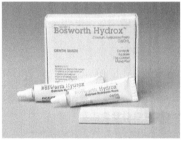
(b)

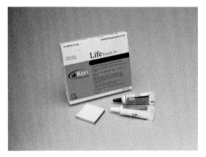
(c)

Figure 9.1 (a) Dycal® – Dentsply. (b) Hydrox™ – Bosworth. (c) Life – Kerr.

ENDODONTIC MATERIALS

Manipulation (Figures 9.2a–9.2c)

Wearing personal protective equipment:
 Two-paste system:

Step 1

- Dispense equal volume of both catalyst and base onto a waxed paper pad according to the manufacturer's instructions (use sparingly as not much material is needed)
- Do not allow the two pastes to touch as this will prematurely initiate the setting reaction
- Ensure that the correct caps are replaced on the appropriate tube to prevent cross-contamination of the base and catalyst

Step 2

- Mix pastes together in a circular motion until a homogeneous colour is achieved (10–15 seconds)

Step 3

- Pass the material to the operator along with a calcium hydroxide applicator for application
- Have some gauze at hand to wipe the calcium hydroxide applicator in between applications

Step 4

- Receive the calcium hydroxide applicator from the operator

Step 5

- Wipe any excess material from the spatula

Step 6

- Dispose of the paper mixing pad in the contaminated waste bin

Light-cured system:

Step 1

- Dispense material or attach new syringe tip

ENDODONTIC MATERIALS

Step 2

- Pass the material to the operator with a calcium hydroxide applicator for application, or pass syringe
- Have some gauze at hand to wipe instrument in between applications

Step 3

- Receive the calcium hydroxide applicator from the operator
- Light cure the calcium hydroxide and extend the amber light protection shield to protect the eyes of the operator and assistant

Step 4

- Wipe excess material from the calcium hydroxide applicator

Step 5

- Dispose of the syringe tip and or waxed paper pad in the contaminated waste

Mixing time

- Two-paste system – 10 to 15 seconds, light cured and no mixing required

Setting time

- Two-paste system – 1.5 to 2.5 minutes, light-curing material – immediately upon polymerisation

Instruments and materials used in set-up

- Calcium hydroxide material
- Waxed paper pad
- Mixing spatula
- Calcium hydroxide applicator
- Gauze

For light curing:

- Curing light
- Amber light protection shield

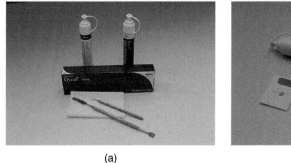
(a)

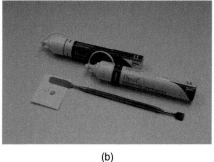
(b)

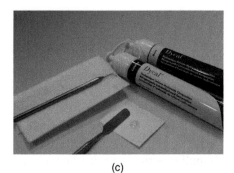
(c)

Figure 9.2 (a) Calcium hydroxide set-up. (b) Calcium hydroxide dispensed. (c) Calcium hydroxide homogenous mix.

MINERAL TRIOXIDE AGGREGATE

Mineral Trioxide Aggregate (MTA) is an endodontic cement that is biocompatible and hydrophilic. It is a powder that is mixed with distilled water.

Material constituents/composition

- Tricalcium oxide
- Silicate oxide
- Bismute oxide

Properties

- Sets in a wet environment
- Setting time is 3–4 hours

ENDODONTIC MATERIALS

- Often referred to as the 'gold standard'
- Placed in oral cavity with an amalgam carrier

Advantages

- Biocompatible
- Antimicrobial
- Hydrophilic properties
- Sealing properties
- Radiopaque

Disadvantages

- Expensive
- Difficult manipulation
- Powder sensitive to humidity – the cap must be replaced immediately after dispensing

Indications for use

Indications
- Sealant in endodontics (perforation of root canal)
- Apexification (non-surgical root canal treatment)
- Repair of root perforations during endodontics
- Direct pulp capping
- Pulpotomy
- Apexogenesis (non-surgical root canal treatment)

Trade names

Trade name	Manufacturer
ProRoot	Dentsply

Manipulation (Figures 9.3a–9.3c)

Wearing personal protective equipment:

Step 1

- Dispense one scoop of MTA and one drop of distilled water on glass slab
- Ensure cap of powder is replaced immediately after dispensing as it is sensitive to humidity

Step 2

- Mix powder and water together with a Weston spatula until a homogenous mixture is achieved (mixing time is 30 seconds)
- The final mixture should resemble wet sand

Step 3

- Fill amalgam carrier and pass to operator to condense in desired location

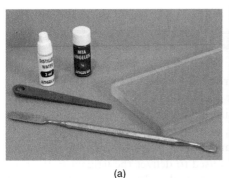
(a)

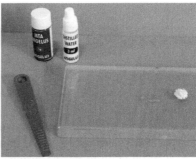
(b)

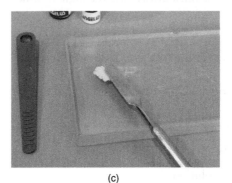
(c)

Figure 9.3 (a) MTA set-up. (b) MTA dispensed. (c) MTA mixed.

ENDODONTIC MATERIALS

Step 4

- Clean and disinfect surface and dispose of excess material in the con-taminated waste bin

Mixing time

- 30 seconds

Setting time

- Initial: 10 minutes; Final: 15 minutes

Instruments and materials used in set-up

- MTA material
- Glass slab
- Weston spatula
- Amalgam carrier
- Dappen dish

IRRIGANTS AND LUBRICANTS

Irrigants and lubricants are used during endodontic treatment to flush and disturb debris from the root canal, for disinfection of the root canal, and other functions. A variety of lubricants and irrigations are used. The operator should choose a solution that is an effective, non-toxic lubricant and which has the ability to flush and break down organic debris from the canal and disinfect it. A disposable blunt-needle syringe is used to deliver the irrigant to the root canal. The dental nurse must always use the high-volume suction during canal irrigation.

Material constituents/composition

The following solutions may be used for irrigation in endodontics:

- Sodium hypochlorite
- Chlorhexidine gluconate
- Local anaesthetic solution
- Saline

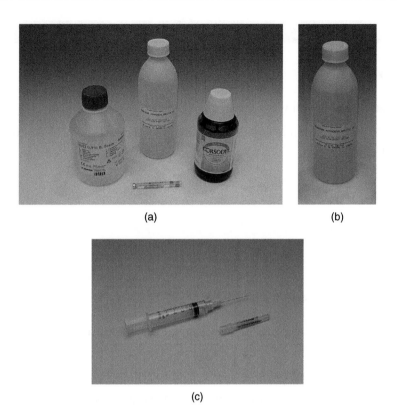

(a)   (b)

(c)

Figure 9.4 (a) Irrigation solutions. (b) Sodium hypochlorite solution. (c) Luer lock syringe with blunt needle for dispensing.

Properties of irrigation solutions (Figure 9.4a)

Solution	Disinfection properties	Ability to break down organic debris	Ability to flush debris	Non-toxic
Sodium hypochlorite	Yes	Yes	Yes	No
Chlorhexidine gluconate (0.2% solution)	Yes	No	Yes	Yes
Local anaesthetic solution	No	No	Yes	Yes
Saline	No	No	Yes	Yes

Sodium hypochlorite is the best choice for irrigation/lubricant as it satisfies most of the desired properties as stated above.

ENDODONTIC MATERIALS

SODIUM HYPOCHLORITE (NaOCl)

Properties

- Dilute solution with water (ratio of 1:1)
- 1–5% concentration of sodium hypochlorite is acceptable for dental irrigation

Advantages

- Widely available
- Cheap

Disadvantages

- Tissue irritant – *must* be used in conjunction with a rubber dam and a high-volume suction
- Must wear personal protective equipment during use
- Ensure patient and operator are wearing safety glasses during use
- Will damage clothing, if comes in contact

Indications and contraindications for use

Indications
- For use with endodontic procedures to irrigate, break down, lubricate, disinfect and flushout debris within the root canal

Contraindications
- Sodium hypochlorite is a tissue irrigant and must not be used without a rubber dam in place

Manipulation

Wearing personal protective equipment:

Step 1

- Check concentration of sodium hypochlorite solution

- Dispense sodium hypochlorite into a disposable cup (you will need to draw up solution multiple times; it is important for infection control purposes to use a disposable cup)

Step 2

- Dilute sodium hypochlorite solution with water to a concentration of 1–5% (usually 1:1 mixture with water)

Step 3

- Use a disposable syringe (e.g. Luer lock) with a blunt side loading needle (e.g. Luer lock) to draw up solution
- Care must be taken to avoid spillages

Step 4

- Pass to the operator extending the plunger of the syringe first (leave the cap on the syringe to pass)
- Once the syringe is securely passed to the operator, the cap may be removed

Step 5

- During irrigation use the high-volume suction to evacuate the used solution

Step 6

- Repeat steps 3–5 as needed

Step 7

- Dispose of the used solution down the sink and dispose of the used syringe in the sharps bin
- Operator to dispose of syringe and needle. If recapping of needle is necessary, do so using the one-handed bayonette technique (Figures 9.4b–9.4c)

Instruments and materials used in set-up

- Irrigation solution

- Disposable syringe (e.g. Luer lock)
- Blunt needle (side loading endodontic, e.g. Luer lock syringe)
- Disposable cup

CHELATING AGENT (CUSTOM LUBRICANT)

A **chelating agent/custom lubricant** may be indicated for use with an endodontic irrigant.

Material constituents/composition

- Ethylene diamine tetra acetic acid (EDTA)

Properties

- Available in gel, liquid and paste forms
- Used for canal irrigation; it softens the canal walls to allow easy negotiation of the root canal

Indications for use

Indications
- To allow easier manipulation and instrumentation of the canal where indicated

Trade names

Trade name	Manufacturer
EDTA Solution (Figure 9.5a)	Pulpdent
File-Rite™ (Figure 9.5b)	Pulpdent
Glyde	Dentsply
RC Prep™ (Figure 9.5c)	Premier products
RC Prep™ Microdose (Figure 9.5d, 9.5e)	Premier products

ENDODONTIC MATERIALS

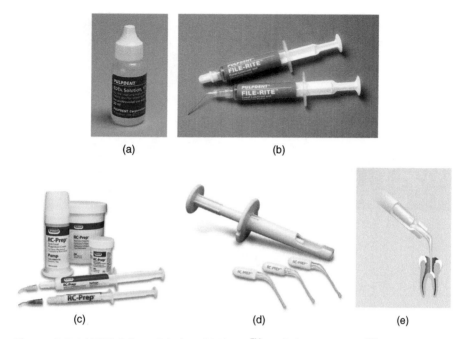

Figure 9.5 (a) EDTA Solution Pulpdent. (b) File-Rite™ – Pulpdent. (c) RC-Prep™ – Premier Dental. (d, e) RC-Prep™ Microdose – Premier Dental.

Manipulation

There is no mixing required for chelating materials.

Figures 9.6(a)–9.6(c) depict RCPrep™ being placed in the canal.

Instruments and materials used in set-up

- Chelating agent
- Dispensing instrument – dropper or spatula
- Paper mixing pad
- Finger or rotary instruments

ENDODONTIC MATERIALS

ENDODONTIC MATERIALS

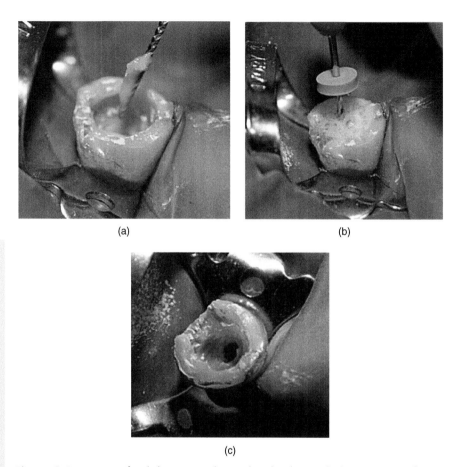

(a)   (b)

(c)

Figure 9.6 Depiction of a chelating agent being placed in the canal (photos courtesy of Premier Dental).

ROOT CANAL OBTURATION

Once pulpal tissue, debris and bacteria have been removed (extirpated) from the root canal by cleaning and shaping, **obturation** (filling the root canal with a material following extirpation of the pulpal tissue) may commence. All root canals are shaped differently. Filling materials must be adaptable to the different canal shapes. Gutta percha is the most commonly used material for obturation. It is used in conjunction with a root canal sealant to fill the canal.

Gutta percha

Material constituents/composition

Two forms of gutta percha are available:

1. α form

- Trans-polyisoprene (isomer of natural rubber)

2. β form

- Trans-polyisoprene (isomer of natural rubber)
- Zinc oxide and additives
- Additives (colours, resins, waxes, metallic salts and antioxidants)

Properties

- Less elastic and more brittle than natural rubber
- The α form is used with heat-softened gutta percha (pellets and gun system)

The β form is used with cold compaction of gutta percha (cones or points used with lateral condensation)

- The β form is the most commonly used and is available in both ISO (International Organisation for Standardisation) standard and non-standardised forms

ISO standardised gutta percha:

- Known as 'standardised' gutta percha
- Follows the International Organisation for Standardisation (ISO) classification of endodontic K files
- e.g. A size 30 gutta percha point should fit a space that was prepared with a size 30 endondontic K file
- Referred to as a master point

Non-standardised gutta percha:

- Known as 'non-standardised' gutta percha
- Used to fill the coronal two-thirds after the placement of the master point (standardised gutta percha)
- May be supplied as fine, medium, etc

Advantages

- Flexible
- Dimensionally stable

- Non-toxic
- Retreatable in the event of root canal failure
- The β form has antibacterial characteristics (contains zinc oxide)

Disadvantages

- Shrinkage on cooling
- Technique sensitive

Indications and contraindications for use

Indications
- Used for the obturation of root canals
- Can be used thermoplasticised or in cold compaction forms
- Cold compaction of gutta percha is carried out in conjunction with a canal sealant

Contraindications
- Patients with a latex allergy

Trade names

Available from many manufacturers.

Manipulation

No manipulation is needed with gutta percha – see page 163 for an example of an obturation technique (there are many techniques) and the materials used in conjunction with obturation (Figure 9.7).

ROOT CANAL SEALER/SEALANT

Material constituents/composition

Available in pastes containing:

- Zinc oxide eugenol
- Calcium hydroxide

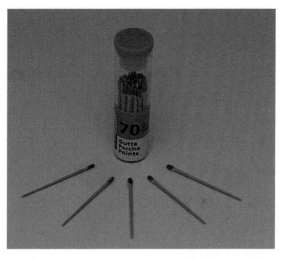

Figure 9.7 Gutta percha.

Other

- Silicone
- Resin

Calcium hydroxide and zinc oxide eugenol based products are the most commonly used and will be discussed in this chapter.

ROOT CANAL SEALER BASED ON CALCIUM HYDROXIDE

Material constituents/composition

- Constituents vary between manufacturers' products; the following constituents are specific to Sealapex (Kerr, 2009):

Base	Catalyst
N-ethyl toluene solfanamide resin	Isobutyl salicylate resin
Fumed silica (silicon dioxide)	Fumed silica (silicon dioxide)
Zinc oxide	Bismuth trioxide
Calcium oxide	Titanium dioxide pigment

ENDODONTIC MATERIALS

Properties

- Fills voids and canal irregularities
- Used to lubricate gutta percha cones and points during lateral condensation
- Aids in retention of gutta percha points
- Maintains a seal around the gutta percha

Advantages

- Long working time (20+ minutes)
- High pH (alkaline)
- Biocompatible/antimicrobial

Disadvantages

- High solubility (not much more soluble than the zinc oxide eugenol type)

Indications and contraindications for use

Indications
- Used in conjunction with gutta percha material

Contraindications
- Unsuitable for use on its own (bulk placement) due to its contractibility and solubility

Trade names

Trade name	Manufacturer
Sealapex – Ca(OH)$_2$ (Figure 9.8)	Kerr
Tubliseal – ZOE	Kerr

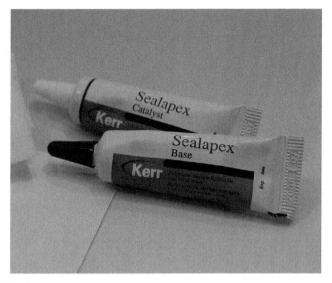

Figure 9.8 Sealapex – Kerr.

Manipulation (Figures 9.9a–9.9c)

Two-paste system:

Step 1

- Dispense equal volume of both catalyst and base onto a waxed paper pad according to the manufacturer's instructions
- Do not allow the two pastes to touch as this will prematurely initiate the setting reaction
- Ensure that the correct caps are replaced on the appropriate tubes to prevent cross contamination of the base and catalyst

Step 2

- Mix pastes together in a circular motion until a homogeneous colour is achieved (10–15 seconds)

Step 3

- Pass the material to the operator on a waxed paper pad along with gutta percha material

Step 4

- Wipe any excess material from the spatula

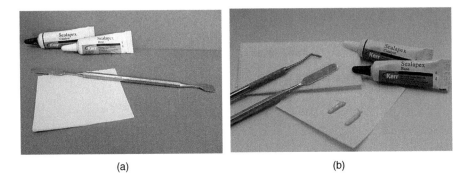

(a)   (b)

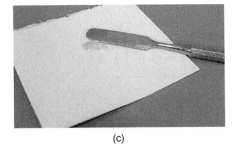

(c)

Figure 9.9 (a) Root canal sealer set-up. (b) Root canal sealer dispensed. (c) Root canal sealer mixed.

Step 6

- Dispose of the paper mixing pad in the contaminated waste bin

See page 163 for an example of an obturation technique (there are many techniques) and the materials used in conjunction with obturation.

Instruments and materials used in set-up

- Root canal sealer
- Waxed paper mixing pad
- Weston spatula

ZINC OXIDE EUGENOL BASED ROOT CANAL SEALER

Material constituents/composition

- Constituents vary between manufacturers' products

Tubliseal is available as a two-paste system and has the following constituents:

Base	Catalyst
Zinc oxide	Eugenol
Oleo resin	Polymerised resin
Bismuth trioxide	Annidalin
Thymol iodide	
Oils	
Waxes	

Other products are available in two-paste systems and powder and liquid systems.

Properties

- Fills voids and canal irregularities
- Used to lubricate gutta percha cones and points during lateral condensation
- Cements gutta percha points in place
- Maintains a seal around the gutta percha

Advantages

- Bacteriocidal properties
- Better adhesion to canal walls than calcium hydroxide based products
- More radiopaque than calcium hydroxide based products (depending on additives)

Disadvantages

- Some zinc oxide eugenol based canal sealers have silver constituents, which can stain dentine

Indications and contraindications for use

Indications
- Used in conjunction with gutta percha material

Contraindications

- Unsuitable for use on its own (bulk placement) due to high shrinkage and solubility

Manipulation

Two-paste system:

Step 1

- Dispense equal volumes of both catalyst and base onto a waxed paper pad according to the manufacturer's instructions
- Do not allow the two pastes to touch as this will prematurely initiate the setting reaction
- Ensure that the correct caps are replaced on the appropriate tube to prevent cross-contamination of the base and catalyst

Step 2

- Mix pastes together in a circular motion until a homogeneous colour is achieved (10–15 seconds)

Step 3

- Pass the material to the operator on a waxed paper pad along with gutta percha material

Step 4

- Wipe any excess material from the spatula

Step 5

- Dispose of the paper mixing pad in the contaminated waste bin

See page 163 for an example of one technique of obturation and materials used in conjunction with obturation.

Instruments and materials used in set-up

- Root canal sealer
- Waxed paper mixing pad
- Weston spatula

- Spreader

- Spiral filler/spiral lentulo

*THE FOLLOWING IS AN EXAMPLE OF AN OBTURATION TECH-
NIQUE, THERE ARE MANY DIFFERING TECHNIQUES; TECHNIQUE IS
DICTATED BY TREATMENT AND THE OPERATOR'S PREFERENCE.*

Wearing personal protective equipment:

Step 1

- Place radiograph(s) on the x-ray viewer

- Local anaesthetic is administered

- The tooth is isolated using a rubber dam

Step 2

- The pulp chamber is accessed through the occlusal (posterior teeth) or
  the lingual (anterior teeth) surface using the turbine/high-speed handpiece and bur

- Evacuate the oral cavity using the high-volume suction

Step 3

- Pass the operator an endodontic broach to extirpate the pulp tissue.
  These instruments must be passed safely using an endondontic block
  or other method that ensures the safety of the patient and staff

- Use an endodontic block to pass endodontic broaches, endodontic K
  files or other finger instruments chance of percutaneous injury

- Gates-Gliden drills and the turbine/low speed handpiece are used to
  enlarge the coronal third of the canal

Step 4

- The operator will use endodontic K files (or equivalent) to smooth and
  shape the canal

- A periapical radiograph is taken to indicate the 'working length' of
  the canal with the endodontic K file (or equivalent) in place (an apex
  locator may also be used to aid in finding this measurement)

- This will be a measurement in millimetres with a coronal reference
  point that must be recorded (if treating a multi-rooted tooth, there will

ENDODONTIC MATERIALS

be a working length and reference point for each root; ensure these measurements and reference points are clearly recorded)

- Measure the endodontic K files (or equivalent) to the working lengths, using rubber stops to mark the measurements
- The operator will continue to smooth and shape the canal at this length (which is 0.5 mm of the maximum constriction point of the root)

Step 5

- Irrigation solution of the operator's choice will be used throughout the procedure to flush, lubricate, disinfect and remove debris from the canal
- The dental nurse must have the irrigant, syringe and blunt needle prepared
- Use the high-volume suction for evacuation during irrigation

Step 6

- The operator's preference and the individual treatment will determine if obturation can continue at this appointment, or if the patient must return at a later date
- If the patient needs to return at a later date, a cotton pellet and temporary restoration are placed over the exposed pulp canal
- If continuing with the procedure, continue to step 7

Step 7

- If the operator is satisfied that the canal is completely cleaned, shaped and irrigated, a master point (gutta percha cone) that corresponds to the same-sized endodontic K file is placed
- A periapical radiograph with the master point in place is taken to ensure the desired length has been achieved

Step 8

- Obturation commences with the canal being dried with paper points
- Pass the operator a paper point loaded in locked college tweezers
- Use two pairs of college tweezers (load one while the operator dries the canal with the other)
- Repeat until the canal is dry

Step 9

- Dispense equal volumes of root canal sealer both catalyst and base onto a paper mixing pad according to the manufacturer's instructions
- Do not allow the two pastes to touch
- Ensure that the correct caps are replaced on the appropriate tubes to prevent cross-contamination of the base and catalyst

Step 10

- Mix pastes together in a circular motion until a homogeneous colour is achieved (10–15 seconds)

Step 11

- The operator may use a spiral filler/spiral lentulo in conventional/slow handpiece, coated in the root canal sealer to coat the walls of the pulp chamber
- Pass the root canal sealer to the operator along with a master point locked into the college tweezers

Step 12

- Receive college tweezers and pass the operator a spreader (finger or hand instrument)

Step 13

- Load college tweezers with an accessory point and coat with a thin layer of root canal sealer
- Pass to the operator

Step 14

- Repeat steps 12 and 13 until the root canal is completely filled with gutta percha

Step 15

- Wipe the excess material from the spatula and instruments with care

Step 16

- The operator will heat an instrument and remove the excess gutta percha from the tooth

ENDODONTIC MATERIALS

Step 17

- Prepare the desired material for the operator to complete the tooth restoration

Step 18

- Dispose of the paper mixing pad in the contaminated waste bin

Mixing time

- Dependent on the type of material used (check the manufacturer's instructions)

Working time

- Dependent on the type of material used (check the manufacturer's instructions)

Setting time

- Dependent on the type of material used (check the manufacturer's instructions)

Instruments and materials used in set-up

- Gutta percha
- Root canal sealer
- Paper mixing pad
- Weston spatula
- Irrigation solution
- Irrigation syringe
- Blunt needle
- Disposable cup

FURTHER READING

Abedi, H.R. and Ingle, J.I. (2005). Mineral trioxide aggregate: a review of a new cement. *Journal of California Dental* Association, 23(12): 36–39.

ENDODONTIC MATERIALS

Kerr, CA. (2009). *Sealapex (base and catalyst) Material Safety Data Sheet.* Available at http://www.sybronendo.com/msds/sybronendo/us/english/SealapexBaseandCatalyst. pdf (Accessed: 12 February 2009).

Kerr, CA. (2006) *Life Catalyst Paste Material Safety Data Sheet.* Available online at http://www.kerrtotalcare.com/msds/kerrdental/us/english/LifeCatalystPaste.pdf (Accessed 12 March 2009).

Kerr, CA. (2006) *Life Base Paste Material Safety Data Sheet.* Available online at http://www.kerrtotalcare.com/msds/kerrdental/us/english/LifeCatalystPaste.pdf (Accessed 12 March 2009).

Chapter 10
Periodontal dressings

A **periodontal dressing** is a 'bandage' that is placed over a surgical site once haemorrhaging has been controlled. The area where the periodontal dressing is to be placed must be relatively dry for the dressing to adhere.

Material constituents/composition

- Available in two-paste, single-paste and light-curable forms
- Zinc oxide eugenol and non-eugenol forms are available

Properties

- Non-toxic

Advantages

- Easily manipulated

Disadvantages

- Material is very sticky (Vaseline must be used on gloves when rolling into a rope to avoid it sticking)

Indications and contraindications for use

Indications
- To promote healing after periodontal treatment, gingivectomies and surgical procedures
- To protect the wound area
- To hold a periodontal flap in position
- To improve the patient's comfort

Contraindications
- Some patients have reported a sensitivity to the material

PERIODONTAL DRESSINGS

Trade names

Trade name	Manufacturer
Coe-Pak™ (Figure 10.1a)	GC America
Perio Care (Figure 10.1b)	Pulpdent

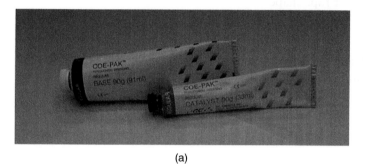
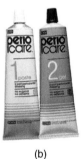

(a)   (b)

Figure 10.1 (a) Coe-pak™ – GC America. (b) Perio Care Pulpdent.

Manipulation (Figures 10.2a–10.2g)

Two-paste system

Wearing personal protective equipment:

Step 1

- When the haemorrhaging from the surgery is under control and on instruction from the operator, extrude equal lengths of both pastes onto a paper mixing pad (approximately 2 inches for each quadrant)

- If there is a paper mixing pad included with the material, use it for mixing

- Ensure that the two pastes do not touch prior to mixing as this will cause the material to prematurely set

Step 2

- Spatulate the material together with a wooden-handled spatula or the spatula supplied by the manufacturer until a homogenous mix (i.e. the material has a uniform colour) is achieved

Step 3

- Using the edge of the spatula, gather the material together and form a cylindrical or rope shape

Step 4

- Prior to handling, lubricate gloves with Vaseline or lanolin and test the periodontal dressing for tackiness (usually takes 2–3 minutes)

Step 5

- Pass the operator some sterile gauze to wipe and dry the area gently

Step 6

- Form the periodontal dressing into small ropes (or desired shapes) for the operator (slightly larger than the area of the wound)

Step 7

- Receive the gauze from the operator and extend the periodontal dressing material on the paper mixing pad

Step 8

- The operator will apply the periodontal dressing so that approximately one-third of the clinical crown is covered as well as the wound
- Prepare and pass the operator a damp cotton tipped applicator. The operator may use it to apply slight pressure to the dressing to adapt it to the interproximal areas
- Pass the operator a hand instrument to remove/trim the excess material
- The periodontal dressing must not be over-packed as excess material tends to break away, causing dislodgement of the dressing

Step 9

- Wipe excess material from the spatula and dispose of the paper mixing pad and excess material into the contaminated waste bin

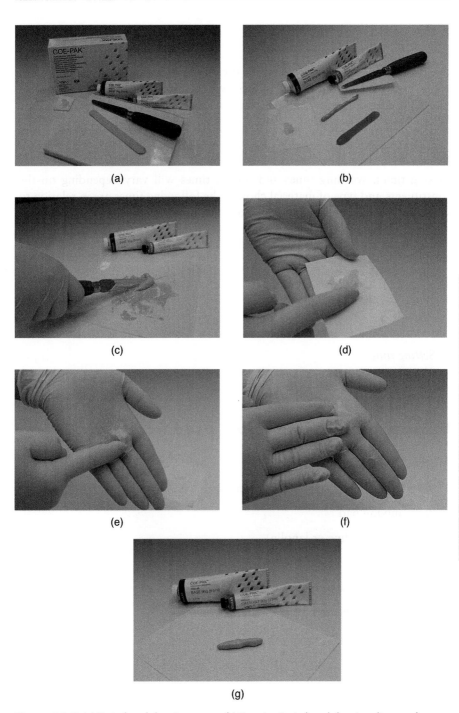

Figure 10.2 (a) Periodontal dressing set-up. (b) Step 1 – Periodontal dressing dispensed. (c) Step 2 – Commencement of mix. (d–f) Step 4 – coating gloves with Vaseline. (g) Step 6 – roll material into a rope.

Step 10
  Post-operative instructions (in relation to the periodontal dressing):

  - Explain to the patient that the dressing is intended to stay in place until their next appointment where it will be removed; and if it is displaced prematurely, they should telephone the surgery

  - Try to eat on the opposite side of the dressing and avoid hard foods that may cause the dressing to be displaced

Mixing times, working times and setting times will vary depending on the constituents and type of material chosen; the following times are in relation to a two-paste non-eugenol zinc oxide paste (regular set).

Mixing time

  - 35–40 seconds

Working time

  - 10–15 minutes

Setting time

  - 30 minutes

Instruments and materials used in set-up

- Periodontal dressing material
- Wooden-handled spatula or manufacturer's supplied spatula
- Paper mixing pad
- Lubricant (Vaseline or lanolin)
- Sterile gauze
- Cotton-tipped applicator
- Hand instrument used for trimming the material

Chapter 11
Dental impression materials

Impressions are used in the dental surgery to produce accurate (varying degrees of accuracy) negative reproductions of the patients' teeth, surrounding tissues and dental arches. Casts (positive reproductions) are created from dental impressions and are used to fabricate various dental prostheses. Different types of impression materials are available. Technique, accuracy, taste, ease of manipulation, cost, dimensional stability and the operator's preference will dictate the choice of impression materials (Figure 11.1).

Impression materials are loaded into trays in their initial low viscous form (with the exception of impression compound) and then placed in the patient's mouth. The impression material will set chemically or physically and then may be removed from the mouth for use extra orally.

TYPES OF IMPRESSION TRAYS

Impression trays are used to hold the impression material, allowing the operator to place it into the patients' mouth. They may be perforated for better retention of the impression material. Different types of impression trays are shown and listed below with their distinguishing characteristics. Adhesives may be indicated with the use of some trays to aid in the retention of the impression materials.

1. Edentulous metal perforated impression trays (Figure 11.2a)

   - For use with edentulous patients

   - Autoclavable

   - Available in different sizes

   - Not easily adapted

   - Available in perforated and non-perforated trays

   - May be used in conjunction with an adhesive

2. Edentulous plastic perforated impression trays (Figure 11.2b)

   - For use with edentulous patients

   - Single use

   - Available in different sizes

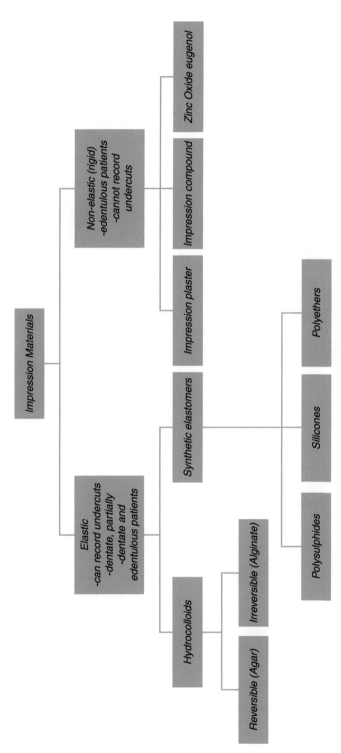

Figure 11.1 Impression material classification (elastic properties).

DENTAL IMPRESSION MATERIALS

DENTAL IMPRESSION MATERIALS

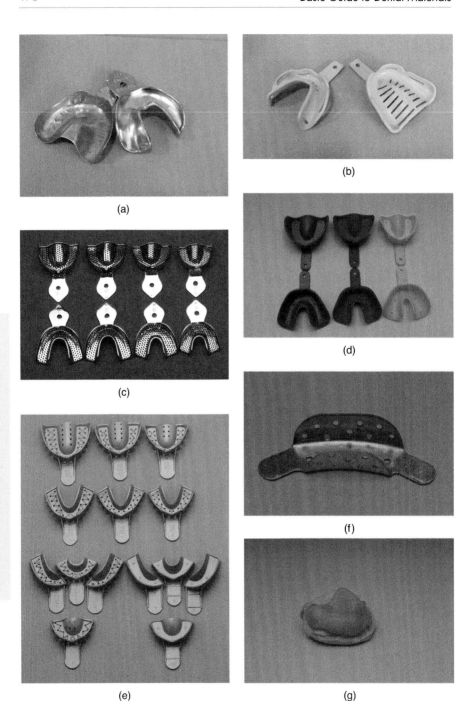

Figure 11.2 (a) Edentulous metal impression trays. (b) Edentulous plastic perforated impression trays. (c) Dentate metal perforated impression trays. (d, e) Dentate plastic perforated 'stock' trays. (f) Universal sectional impression trays. (g) Custom/special tray.

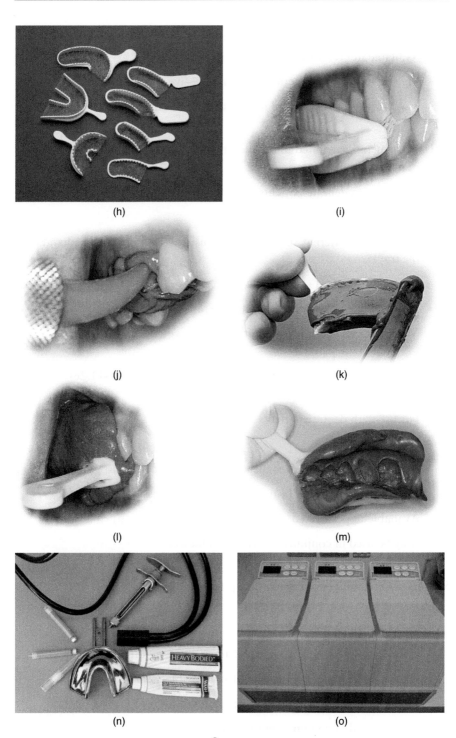

(h)

(i)

(j)

(k)

(l)

(m)

(n)

(o)

Figure 11.2 (*Continued*) (h–m) Triple tray®. (n, o) Set up for Reversible Hydrocolloid Impression Material.

- Easily adapted using a heat source and/or impression compound
- Available in perforated and non-perforated trays
- May be used in conjunction with an adhesive
- May have a separate metal handle that is autoclavable

3. Dentate metal perforated impression trays (Figure 11.2c)

- For use with dentate patients
- Autoclavable
- Available in different sizes (the size is usually engraved on the handle of the tray)
- Not easily adapted
- Available in perforated and non-perforated trays
- May be used in conjunction with an adhesive

4. Dentate plastic perforated impression trays (Figures 11.2d–11.2e)

- For use with dentate patients
- Single use
- Available in different sizes (usually denoted by colours)
- Easily adapted using a heat source and/or impression compound
- Available in perforated and non-perforated trays
- May be used in conjunction with an adhesive

5. Universal sectional impression tray (Figure 11.2f)

- For use with dentate patients
- Used for impressions of a specific areas of the mouth
- Easily adapted as it is fabricated from flexible metal
- Available in perforated and non-perforated trays
- May be used in conjunction with an adhesive

6. Custom/ special tray (Figure 11.2g)

- Fabricated from a plaster model of the patient's dentate or edentulous arch
- Fabricated from an acrylic material
- Single use
- May be used in conjunction with an adhesive

7. Triple tray® (Figures 11.2h–11.2m)

- Used to take an impression of both arches simultaneously
- Fabricated from a combination of plastic and flexible webbing material
- Different sizes available
- Single use
- May be used in conjunction with an adhesive

DECONTAMINATION OF IMPRESSIONS

It is necessary to decontaminate impressions to prevent cross-contamination. Once an impression is removed from the patient's mouth, the following procedure should be undertaken:

Wearing personal protective equipment:

- Inspect the dental impression for blood and/or debris. Wash in a designated sink to remove the same
- The disinfection process will be impeded without adequate removal of blood and/or debris
- Follow the manufacturer's instructions in relation to the immersion of the dental impression in a disinfectant solution for material compatibility and length of immersion
- After impression decontamination, rinse impression in the designated sink
- It is essential that good cross-infection control practices are followed during impression decontamination; avoid contamination of immersion bath and sink. If contamination occurs, disinfect
- Disinfected impressions should be prepared for the laboratory by placing in a sealable bag, taking care to not cross-contaminate the bag. Seal the bag

DENTAL IMPRESSION MATERIALS

- Complete laboratory prescription ensuring that the date, time and solution of disinfectant is recorded

- Staple laboratory prescription to the sealed bag above the seal, taking care to not perforate bag

- Transport to the dental laboratory

When receiving laboratory work, disinfect and rinse prior to inserting into the patient's mouth.

(*Adapted from the Cross Infection Control Policy, Dublin Dental Hospital, 2010.*)

ELASTIC IMPRESSION MATERIALS – HYDROCOLLOID IMPRESSION MATERIALS

A. Reversible Hydrocolloid Impression Material (Agar)

Agar impression materials have been largely replaced by rubber impression materials.

Material constituents/composition

Supplied as a gel in a tube

- Agar
- Borax
- Potassium sulphate
- Alkyl benzoate
- Colours
- Flavours
- Water

Properties

- The material has two forms: sol (fluid) and gel (more viscous)
- Hydrophilic

- Once set to the gel state, given the right temperature, it can be reversed to the liquid (sol) state

Advantages

- Accurate
- High definition
- Easy to manipulate
- Used for hard and soft tissue impressions
- Economical
- Non-toxic
- Non-staining
- Hydrophilic

Disadvantages

- Longer preparation time
- Tears easily
- Long setting time
- Needs to be poured immediately
- Initially expensive to purchase specialised equipment
- Dimensionally unstable
- Claims to be reusable, but due to infection control issues this is not acceptable

Indications and contraindications for use

Indications
- Full-arch impressions
- Quadrant impressions
- Partial denture impressions

Contraindications
- Trays are very bulky and may not be tolerated by certain patients

Trade names

Trade name	Manufacturer
Hydrocolloid Agar Blue	VanR

Manipulation

There is no manipulation needed for agar impression materials, but a special water bath with three compartments (Figure 11.1n) is needed to facilitate the use of this impression material. Care must be taken to ensure that the water bath is not contaminated during use (Figures 11.2n–11.2o).

Mixing time

- There is no mixing needed

Setting time

- 5 minutes

Instruments and materials used in set-up

- Desired impression material
- Syringe, needle
- Impression tray
- Tubing
- Tissue and rinse cup for the patient
- Laboratory bag
- Laboratory prescription
- Special water bath with three compartments

B. Irreversible Hydrocolloid Impression Material (Alginate)

Alginate is one of the most commonly used impression materials in the dental surgery with wide range of uses. It is mixed with water to achieve the desired mixture.

Material constituents/composition

Available in jars, bulk packaging and pre-measured packs. A measuring scoop and water measure are included with the alginate materials.

- Salt of alginic acid
- Trisodium phosphate
- Fillers (diatomaceous earth)
- Colours
- Flavours
- Calcium sulphate dehydrate
- Potassium sulphate

Properties

- Available in regular and fast-set forms
- Dust-free powder
- Working and setting times may be adjusted by increasing or decreasing the temperature of the water (increasing temperature, decreases working and setting times and decreasing temperature increases working and setting times)
- Optimal water temperature is 21°C
- Some materials are available that change colour as they change state; this aids in ensuring that materials are completely set prior to removal from the mouth

Advantages

- Easy to manipulate
- Cheap
- Rapid setting
- Elastic properties make it a suitable material for taking impressions where there are undercuts
- Hydrophilic

DENTAL IMPRESSION MATERIALS

Disadvantages

- Poor dimensional stability

- Models must be poured within one hour and kept moist until poured

- Not as precise as secondary impression materials

- Room temperature and humidity can affect working and setting time of alginate

Indications and contraindications for use

Indications
Impressions for:

- Study models

- Removable partial dentures

- Fabrication of temporary/provisional crowns and bridges

- Fabrication of custom/special trays

- Orthodontic applicances

- Bleaching trays

- Mouth guards

Contraindications
- Not as accurate as other products so they are not suitable for crown and bridge impressions

- Care must be taken when taking impressions of patients with strong gag reflexes

Trade names

Trade name	Manufacturer
Blueprint Cremex	Dentsply
Hydrogum® (Figure 11.3a)	Zhermack
Integra™	Kerr
Jeltrate®	Carson Dental
Kromopan® 100	Kromopan
Xantalgin® Select (Figure 11.3b)	Heraeus

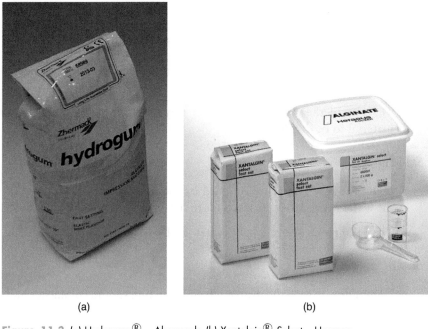

(a)   (b)

Figure 11.3 (a) Hydrogum® – Ahermack. (b) Xantalgin® Select – Heraeus.

Manipulation (Figures 11.4a–11.4k)

Wearing personal protective equipment:

Step 1

- The patient's oral cavity should be free of debris prior to taking alginate impressions

Step 2

- Pass the operator the impression tray (maxillary or mandibular) for try-in (if needed, add impression compound to alter or extend the impression tray)

Step 3

- Ensuring to not cross-contaminate the bottle, use a disposable applicator brush to apply tray adhesive to the impression tray if indicated (it is best practice to dispense some adhesive and then use a disposable brush to apply over the impression tray to avoid contamination)

- Ensure that tray adhesive is painted on the rim area of the impression tray as well as the body

Step 4

- Fluff the alginate in the jar and dispense the alginate powder using the measuring scoop provided by the manufacturer (overfill the scoop from jar and level using a disposable tongue depressor or a sterilised fish tailed spatula)

- The size of the selected impression tray will dictate the amount of material to be dispensed

Step 5

- Using the water measure supplied by the manufacturer, measure out the water needed (this corresponds to the amount of powder dispensed)

- The ideal temperature for the water is $21°C$

Step 6

- Communicate with the dentist when the mixing should commence and add the powder and water

- Mix the powder and water with a stirring motion, using the tip of the spatula

- Turn the bowl on its side in the palm of your hand and rotate the bowl, continuing to mix the material with the wide part of the spatula blade until a homogenous mixture is achieved

Step 7

- Gather the alginate in the bowl and using the blade of the spatula, pick up the material to load the impression tray

Step 8

- Load the impression tray using the spatula

- The mandibular tray is loaded from the lingual using an overlapping technique to ensure the tray is completely filled

- The maxillary tray is filled from the posterior region and material is continuously added with pressure until the tray is full

- Extra impression material may be required for the operator to manually insert in the event that a patient has a high palate

- Leave some excess material on the back of your gloved hand – this is used to check if the material is set after placement in the oral cavity

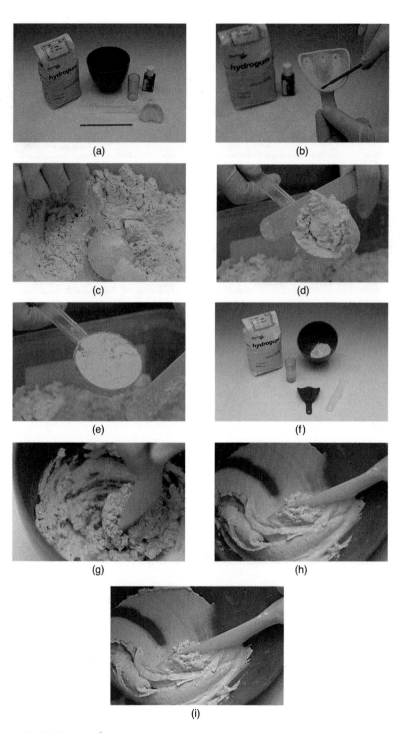

(a)　　　　　　　　　　(b)

(c)　　　　　　　　　　(d)

(e)　　　　　　　　　　(f)

(g)　　　　　　　　　　(h)

(i)

DENTAL IMPRESSION MATERIALS

Figure 11.4 (*Continued*)

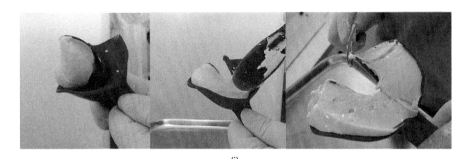

(j)

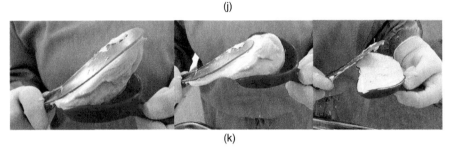

(k)

Figure 11.4 (a) Irreversible Hydrocolloid Impression material set-up. (b) Step 3 – Painting the stock tray with adhesive on an impression tray prior to use. (c–e) Step 4 – dispensing the powder. (f) Step 5 – Water measured out and powder dispensed. (g–i) Step 6 – Material manipulation (spatulation). (j) Step 8 – Loading a mandibular impression tray. (k) Step 8 – Loading a maxillary impression tray.

DENTAL IMPRESSION MATERIALS

Step 9

- Once the impression tray is filled, hand the tray to the operator extending the tray handle first

Step 10

- Remove excess material from spatula and flexible mixing bowl and dispose of in the contaminated waste bin

Disinfect the flexible mixing bowl and fish-tailed spatula.
See section on *Decontamination of impressions.*

Mixing time
  Regular set: 1 minute
  Fast set: 45 seconds

Working time
  Regular set: 3–4.5 minutes
  Fast set: 1.25–2 minutes

Setting time
   Regular set: 1–4.5 minutes
   Fast set: 1–2 minutes

Elastomeric impression materials are widely used in the dental surgery when accuracy of an impression is important. They have good tear resistance and dimensional stability (two advantages over hydrocolloids). Each material has a range of varying viscosities (light, medium and heavy).

A. Polysulphides (Polysulfides) (Rubber Base) Impression Materials

Material constituents/composition

- Supplied in a two-paste system
- Available in low, medium and high viscosity

Base	Catalyst
Polysulphide polymer	Lead dioxide
Reinforcing fillers	Hydrated copper oxide or organic peroxide
Plasticisers	Sulphur
	Dibutyl phthalate

Properties

- The working and setting times are altered with heat and humidity
  - Higher the temperature and humidity, the shorter the working and setting time
  - Lower the temperature and humidity, the longer the working and setting time
- Hydrophilic
- Useful when a long working time is needed

DENTAL IMPRESSION MATERIALS

Advantages

- High accuracy
- Long working time
- Good tear strength
- Low cost

Disadvantages

- Material will stain clothes
- Very unpleasant odour
- Must be used in conjunction with a custom/special tray

Runny consistency

- Long setting time
- Cast must be poured within an hour
- Polysulphides contract upon storage

Indications and contraindications for use

Indications
- Fixed partial denture impressions
- Crown and bridge impressions
- Implant impressions

Contraindications
- Patients with a strong gag reflex

Trade names

Trade name	Manufacturer
Permlastic® (Figure 11.5)	Kerr

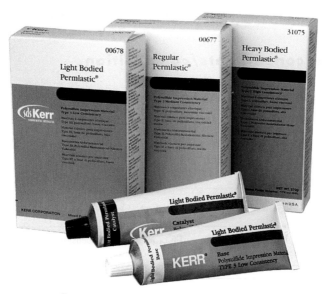

Figure 11.5 Permlastic® – Kerr.

Manipulation

See common manipulation instructions for two-paste dental impressions on page 210.

See section on *Decontamination of impressions*.

Mixing time

- 45–60 seconds

Working time

- 5–7 minutes

Setting time

- 8–12 minutes

Manipulation

See end of this chapter for generic instructions for the manipulation of a two-paste impression material.

B. Silicone Impression Materials

There are two types of silicone impression materials available: condensation and addition or vinyl silicones. They are categorised in relation to the type of reaction responsible for their setting.

CONDENSATION SILICONE IMPRESSION MATERIALS

Material constituents/composition

- Available in two-paste or liquid/paste systems

- Available in light, medium and heavy viscosities as well as a putty

- May be difficult to achieve a uniform mix as base and catalyst pastes are not of the same consistency

Base	Catalyst
Dimethylsiloxane	Tin organic ester suspension
Filler–silica	Alkyl silicate
	Thickening agent

Properties

- Moderate shelf-life
- Moderate tear strength

Advantages

- Accurate
- Easily manipulated
- Fast setting time
- Non-toxic and non-irritant
- Very elastic

Disadvantages

- Setting may be affected by changes in temperature and humidity

- Hydrophobic

- Prone to shrinkage on storage – condensation impressions must be poured up within an hour

Indications and contraindications for use

Indications

- Fixed partial denture impressions

- Inlay and onlay impressions

- Crown and bridge impressions

- Implants

Contraindications

- May cause irritation with some patients

Trade names

Trade name	Manufacturer
Citricon	Kerr
Examix	GC America
Optosil	Bayer
Xantopren® VL Plus (Figure 11.6)	Bayer

Manipulation

See common manipulation instructions for a two-paste or putty dental impression, depending on the type you are mixing.

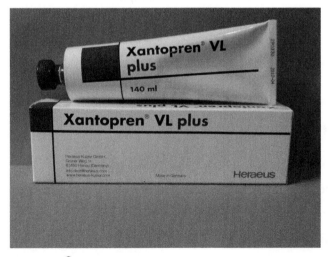

Figure 11.6 Xantopren® VL Plus – Bayer.

See section on *Decontamination of impressions.*

Mixing time

- 45–60 seconds

Working time

- 3 minutes

Setting time

- 6–8 minutes

ADDITION (VINYL) SILICONE IMPRESSION MATERIALS

Material constituents/composition

- Supplied in a two-paste system and automix cartridge system (dispensing gun)
- Available in light, medium and heavy viscosities as well as a putty
- Base and catalyst pastes are the same consistency, which makes manipulation easy
- May be referred to as vinyl polysiloxane impression materials

Base	Catalyst
Polyvinyl siloxane	Polyvinyl siloxane
Filler	Platinum catalyst
Silanol	Filler

Properties

- Accurate
- Good shelf-life
- Dimensionally stable
- Non-toxic and non-irritant
- Moderate tear strength

Advantages

- Accurate
- Easily manipulated
- Range of viscosities
- Fast setting time
- Dimensionally stable – they are not prone to shrinkage on storage – addition silicones can be poured up multiple times. They are more expensive than condensation silicones

Disadvantages

- Setting may be affected by changes in temperature and humidity
- Hydrophobic
- *Powdered latex gloves may retard the setting properties in the putty form of addition silicone impression materials*

Indications and contraindications for use

Indications
- Fixed partial denture impressions
- Inlay and onlay impressions
- Crown and bridge impressions
- Implants

Contraindications
- Using powdered latex gloves during the manipulation of the putty form of material will affect the material properties adversely

Trade names

Trade name	Manufacturer
Express™	3M ESPE
Extrude® (Figure 11.7a)	Kerr
President (Figure 11.7b)	Coltene
Reprosil	Dentsply

DENTAL IMPRESSION MATERIALS

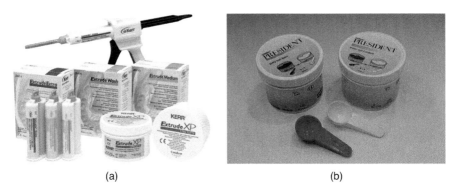

(a)   (b)

Figure 11.7 (a) Extrude® – Kerr. (b) President – Coltene.

Manipulation

See common manipulation instructions for two-paste, putty and Automix gun
dental impressions on page 210.
    See section on *Decontamination of impressions*.

Mixing time

● 45–60 seconds

Working time

● 2–4 minutes

Setting time

● 3–7 minutes

C. Polyether Impression Materials

Polyether impression materials are very rigid (stiff) impression materials.
They have superior mechanical properties to polysulfides and less dimensional
change than silicones.

Material constituents/composition

● Available in a two-paste system, single-mix and an electric mechanical mixer

Base	Catalyst
Polyether	Sulphonic acid ester
Inert filler – silica	Inert filler – silica
Plasticizer	Plasticizer
	Inert oils

DENTAL IMPRESSION MATERIALS

Properties

- Very accurate
- Heat and humidity speed up working and setting times
- Hydrophilic
- Non-toxic
- Good elasticity
- Good dimensional stability
- Low tear strength
- Low setting contraction

Advantages

- Accurate
- Easily manipulated

Disadvantages

- Low tear strength
- Short working time
- Rigid (stiff) material
- May be hard to remove from the mouth due to stiffness

Indications and contraindications for use

Indications
- Crown and bridge impressions
- Partial denture impressions
- Implants

Contraindications
- Due to the rigidity of the material it may be hard to remove from a patient's mouth with mobile teeth

DENTAL IMPRESSION MATERIALS

Trade names

Trade name	Manufacturer
Impregum™ F (Figure 11.8)	3M ESPE
Impregum™ Pentamix™	3M ESPE

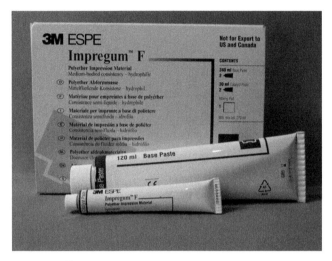

Figure 11.8 Impregum™ F – 3M ESPE.

Manipulation (Figures 11.9a–11.9c)

Wearing personal protective equipment:
Using Impregum™ Pentamix™:

Step 1

- Load impression bag into the cartridge

Step 2

- Insert cartridge into the Pentamix™ machine securely

Step 3

- Place tip onto impression bag

Step 4

- Close lever over impression cartridge

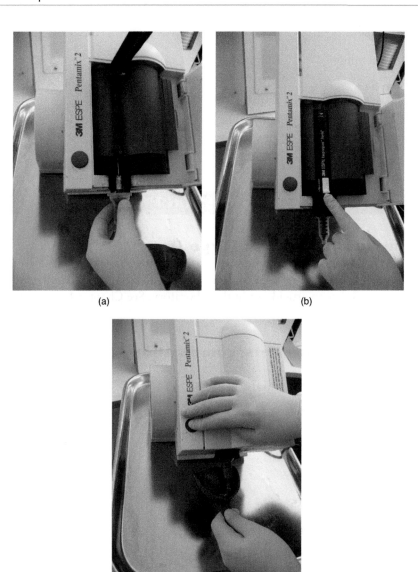

(a)   (b)

(c)

Figure 11.9 (a) Step 3 – Insert mixing tip on to the Pentamix™. (b) Step 4 – Close lever over impression cartridge. (c) Step 5 – Push button to dispense impression material.

Step 5

- Close cover and push button to dispense material

Also see common manipulation instructions for two-paste dental impressions on page 210.

See section on *Decontamination of impressions*.

DENTAL IMPRESSION MATERIALS

Mixing time

- 30–45 seconds

Working time

- 2.5 minutes

Setting time

- 4.5 minutes

NON-ELASTIC (RIGID) IMPRESSION MATERIALS

A. Impression Plaster (Type I)

Impression plaster is rarely used for intra-oral impressions; it is mainly used for mounting casts on an articulator in the laboratory. See Chapter 12 on gypsum materials.

Material constituents/composition

- Calcium sulphate hemihydrate
- Forms calcium sulphate dehydrate when mixed with water
- Available in powder and liquid forms

Properties

- Must be stored in an airtight container
- Manipulation sensitive
- For use with a special tray

Advantages

- Good dimensional stability
- Hydrophilic

Disadvantages

- Brittle
- High fracture rate

Indications and contraindications for use

Indications
* For use in edentulous patients

Contraindications
* If there are any undercuts present

Trade names

Various manufacturers

Manipulation

Water/powder ratio:

* 60 ml water to 100 grams powder

  See Chapter 12 for gypsum manipulation.

Setting time

* 3–5 minutes intra-orally

B. Impression Compound (Compo)

Impression compound is a thermoplastic material used to record a preliminary impression of an edentulous ridge to fabricate a special tray. This material is not often used as there are other superior impression materials. (The stick form of impression compound is still used for the purpose of impression tray extensions and extensions on dentures.)

Material constituents/composition

* Available in cakes, discs, cones and sticks

Constituents of impression compounds vary between manufactures and may contain a combination of the following:

* Resins
* Waxes

- Steric acid
- Fillers
- Colouring agents

Properties

- May be used in conjunction with a wash of zinc oxide eugenol paste to record detail
- Reversible physical reaction

Advantages

- Compatible with die and cast materials

Disadvantages

- Poor dimensional stability (must be poured immediately, within one hour, after recording)
- Need a water bath for softening discs or cakes (allows uniform temperature to be achieved)
- Technique sensitive
- Hot air torch can be used to heat cones or sticks – taking care to not overheat
- Does not record intricate detail

Indications and contraindications for use

Indications
- To take a preliminary impression of an edentulous arch in order to fabricate a special tray

Contraindications
- Where there are undercuts are present

Trade names

Trade name	Manufacturer
Green stick (Figure 11.10)	Kerr
Grey sticks	Kerr
Red cakes (Figure 11.11)	Kerr
Red sticks	Kerr

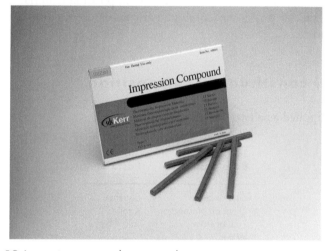

Figure 11.10 Impression compound – green stick.

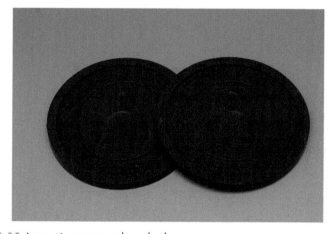

Figure 11.11 Impression compound – red cake.

Manipulation

There is no manipulation required for impression compound. In its initial state it is a rigid material that requires heating in a water bath at 55–60°C. If the water bath is too cold, the material will not be pliable enough; and if the water bath is too hot, the impression compound will become sticky.

C. Zinc Oxide Eugenol

Zinc oxide eugenol paste is mainly used as an impression material in conjunction with a special tray for edentulous patients or used within the patient's existing denture.

Material constituents/composition

Normally supplied as a two-paste system:

Base paste	Paste 2
Zinc oxide	Eugenol
Olive oil, linseed oil	Kaolin
Zinc acetate	Talc (filler)
Water	

Properties

- May be mixed on a paper mixing pad or glass slab
- Petroleum jelly should be applied to the patient's lips and surrounding skin as zinc oxide eugenol paste sticks to the skin's surface

Advantages

- Adapts well to soft tissues
- Low viscosity
- High accuracy
- Inexpensive
- Adheres to impression compound

Disadvantages

- Rigid once set
- Cannot record undercuts
- May leave a taste in the patient's mouth after removal
- May cause a burning sensation in the patient's mouth (it is non-toxic)
- Messy material

Indications and contraindications for use

Indications
- Used as a wash impression material in an impression tray (or patient's denture) for the edentulous patient
- Bite registration

Contraindications
- In areas where undercuts may be present

Trade names

Trade name	Manufacturer
Impression Paste (Figure 11.12)	SSWhite
Kelly's® ZOE	Waterpik
Superpaste™ (Figure 11.13)	Bosworth

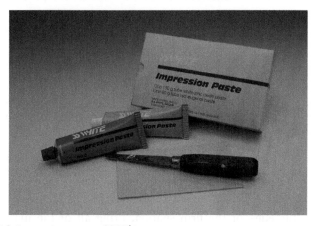

Figure 11.12 Impression paste – SS White.

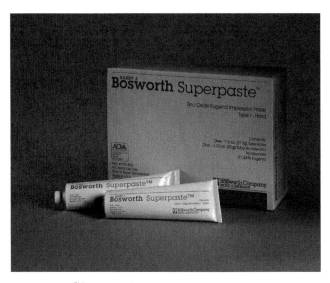

Figure 11.13 Superpaste™ – Bosworth.

Manipulation (Figures 11.14a–11.14e)

Wearing personal protective equipment:

Step 1

- Extrude equal lengths of the two pastes onto a paper mixing pad or glass slab
- The pastes are of different colours, do not let the pastes touch until mixing commences

Step 2

- Using a stiff wooden-handled, stainless steel spatula, spatulate the two pastes together in a circular motion until a uniform colour has been achieved

Step 3

- Using the edge of the firm spatula, bring all of the material to the middle of the paper mixing pad or glass slab

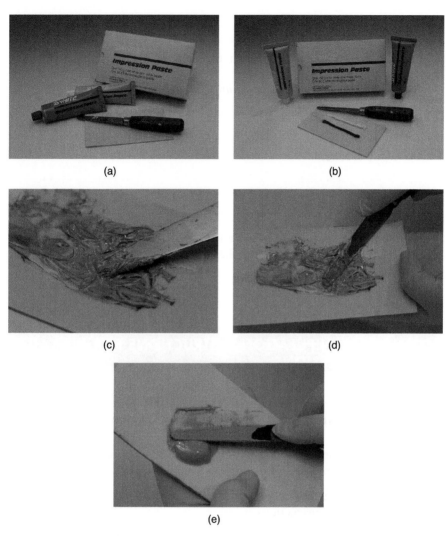

(a)

(b)

(c)

(d)

(e)

Figure 11.14 (a) ZOE impression paste set-up. (b) Step 1 – ZOE impression paste dispensed. (c,d) Step 2 – ZOE manipulation. (e) Step 3 – Gather ZOE in middle of mixing pad.

Step 4

- Cover the impression tray with the material (wash coverage) or extend the mixed material and spatula (handle first) to the operator to cover the impression tray (and receive spatula back)

Step 5

- Clean excess materials from the spatula using orange solvent

DENTAL IMPRESSION MATERIALS

Step 6

- Dispose of paper mixing pad in the contaminated waste bin

See section on *Decontamination of impressions*

Mixing time

- 40–60 seconds

Setting time

- Initial setting in 3–5 minutes and final setting in 10–15 minutes (setting time is shortened with the increase in temperature in the oral cavity)

COMMON MANIPULATION INSTRUCTIONS FOR DENTAL IMPRESSIONS

Preparing an impression tray with tray adhesive prior to loading with impression material

- Prior to the commencement of mixing the impression material the operator will try in the custom/special tray to ensure adequate fit

- Paint the custom/special tray with tray adhesive and allow it to dry as per the manufacturer's instructions

- Ensure that tray adhesive is painted on the rim area of the impression tray as well as the body

- Ensuring to not cross contaminate the bottle, use a disposable applicator brush to apply tray adhesive to the impression tray if indicated (it is best practice to dispense some adhesive and then use a disposable brush to apply the adhesive over the impression tray to avoid contamination). See Figures 11.15 and 11.16

Mixing a two-paste impression material

Wearing personal protective equipment:

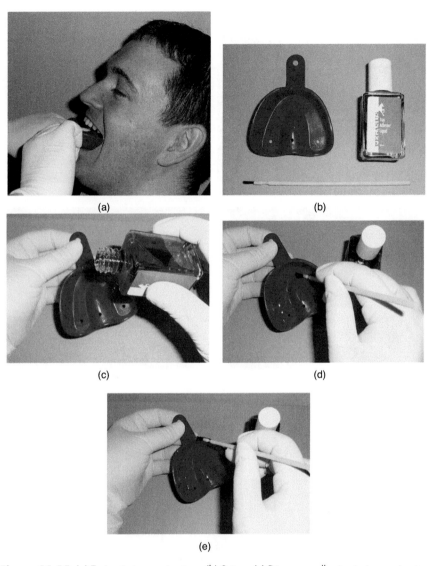

Figure 11.15 (a) Trying in impression tray. (b) Set-up. (c) Dispense adhesive in impression tray using 'no touch' technique to ensure good cross infection control. Disinfect bottle afterwards if necessary. (d, e) Painting adhesive on impression tray ensuring to include rim.

Step 1

- Extrude equal lengths of the two pastes onto a paper mixing pad or glass slab (or if supplied as a liquid and base dispense one drop to one inch of base material)

- The pastes are of different colours, do not let the pastes touch until mixing commences

DENTAL IMPRESSION MATERIALS

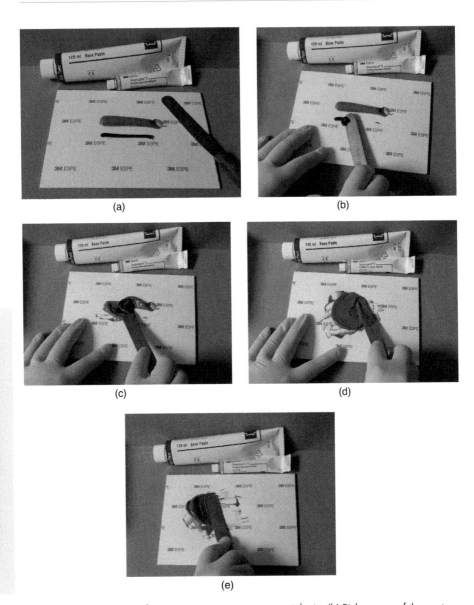

(a)   (b)

(c)   (d)

(e)

Figure 11.16 (a) Set-up for a two-paste impression material mix. (b) Pick up one of the pastes on the side of the spatula for ease of incorporation with the other paste. (c,d) Mixing the impression material. (e) Final homogenous mixture (ensure there are no streaks).

Step 2

- Using a stiff wooden-handled, stainless steel spatula, spatulate the two pastes together in a circular motion until a uniform colour has been achieved

Step 3

- Using the edge of the firm spatula, bring all of the material to the middle of the paper mixing pad or glass slab
- Fill syringe or load impression tray (Figure 11.17)

Step 4

- Clean excess materials from the spatula and syringe

Step 5

- Dispose of paper mixing pad in the contaminated waste bin (Figures 11.17a–11.17k)

Filling a syringe with impression material for dispensing intra-orally

Step 1

- Set up syringe by screwing on dispensing tip and nut. Leave the plunger out of the syringe

Step 2

- Mix two-paste system as explained earlier in this chapter see page 210

Step 3

- Ensuring that the mixed impression material has been gathered in the centre of the waxed paper mixing pad, use the plunger end of the syringe to gather the impression material
- Gathering the impression material is done by making quick strokes on the waxed paper pad while inserting the impression material into the body of the syringe
- Repeat until the desired amount of impression material is loaded into the syringe

Step 4

- Wipe the plunger end of the syringe with a piece of gauze to remove any excess impression material

DENTAL IMPRESSION MATERIALS

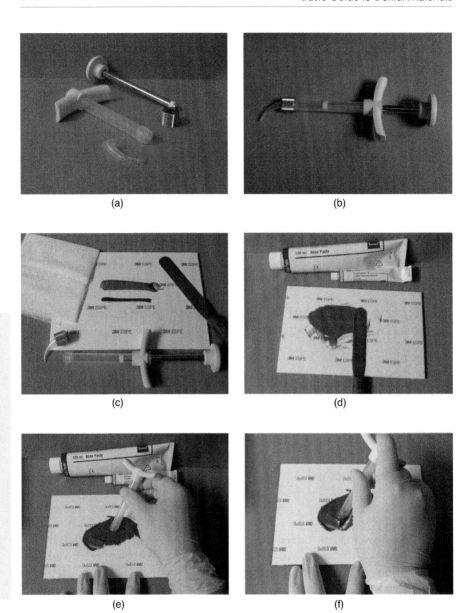

Figure 11.17 (a) Impression syringe pieces. (b) Impression syringe assembled. (c) Impression syringe and material set-up. (d) Homogenous mixture. (e–g) Filling the impression syringe, utilising strokes alike filling an amalgam carrier, until the desired amount is loaded in the syringe.

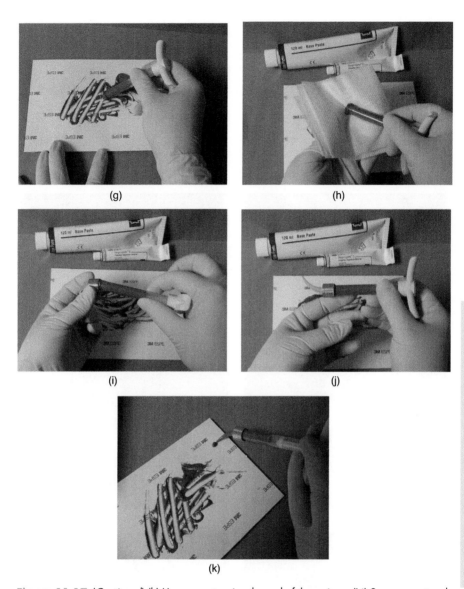

Figure 11.17 (*Continued*) (h) Use gauze to wipe the end of the syringe. (I,j) Screw on nut and syringe tip securely. (k) Expel a small amount of impression material prior to passing to the operator to ensure the syringe is ready for dispensing.

Step 5

- Insert the plunger into the syringe and dispense a small amount of material in preparation, prior to handing it to the operator to dispense intra-orally (Figures 11.18a–11.18k)

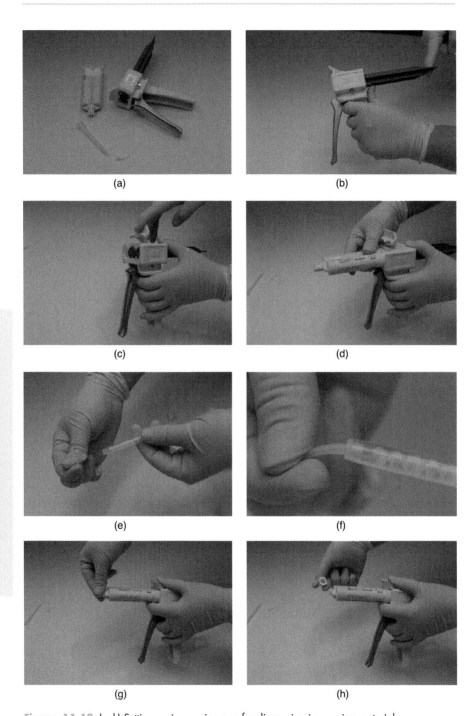

Figure 11.18 (a–k) Setting up impression gun for dispensing impression material.

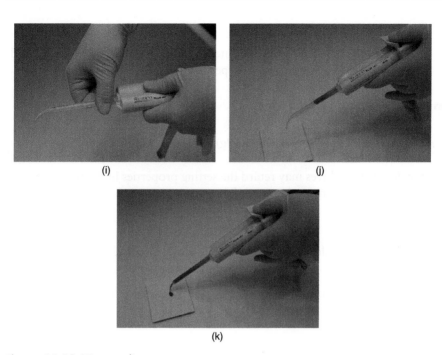

(i)

(j)

(k)

Figure 11.18 (*Continued*)

Setting up an automix cartridge system for impression materials

Step 1

- Pull plunger back

Step 2

- Lift the small plastic cover that holds the impression cartridge in place

Step 3

- Insert impression cartridge

Step 4

- If required, assemble mixing tip (if injecting material intra orally, there is often a small applicator that can be attached to the end of the mixing tip for ease of placement)

Step 5

- Remove the cap from the impression cartridge

Step 6

- Insert the mixing tip onto the impression cartridge with a turning motion

DENTAL IMPRESSION MATERIALS

Step 7

- Extrude a small amount of material onto a waxed paper mixing pad to prepare it for immediate dispensing

Putty manipulation

Putty technique (Figures 11.19a–11.19g)

- Powdered latex gloves may retard the setting properties in the putty form of addition silicone impression materials

Step 1

- Using the colour-coded scoops supplied, dispense one scoop (equal amounts) of both the base and the catalyst

- Place on a waxed paper pad, ensuring they do not touch until ready to use

Step 2

- With clean hands (no gloves) the dental nurse kneads the base and catalyst putties together until a homogenous colour is achieved and loads it into the pre-prepared impression tray. Kneading the putty together should not take more than 30 seconds

Instruments and materials used in set-up (common to all of the above set-ups)

- Desired impression material

- Flexible bowl, paper mixing pad, auto mix gun or machine

- Mixing spatula specific to each material

- Tips for automix gun, syringe or Pentamix™

- Desired type of impression tray

- Tissue and rinse cup for the patient

- Laboratory bag

- Laboratory prescription

Optional

- Tray adhesive and disposable applicator brush

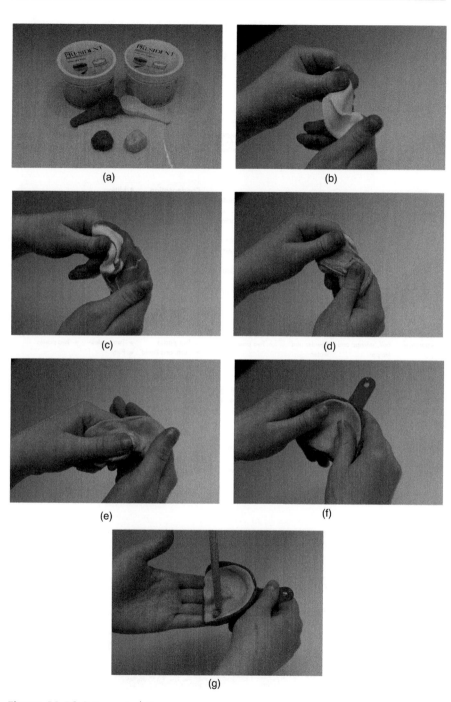

Figure 11.19 Putty manipulation

- Wax and impression compound for altering/extending the impression tray
- Heat source for manipulating plastic stock tray
- Kidney dish
- Orange solvent

SUMMARY CHART OF ELASTIC IMPRESSION MATERIALS

DENTAL IMPRESSION MATERIALS

	Agar	Alginate	Polysulphide	Condensation Silicone	Addition Silicone	Polyether
Use	• Full-arch impressions • Quadrant impressions • Partial denture impressions	• Study models • Partial dentures • Fabrication of temporary crowns and bridges • Fabrication of custom trays • Orthodontic appliances • Bleaching trays • mouthguards	• Fixed partial denture impressions • Crown and bridge impressions • Implant impressions	• Fixed partial denture impressions • Crown and bridge impressions • Implant impressions • Inlay and onlay impressions	• Fixed partial denture impressions • Crown and bridge impressions • Implant impressions • Inlay and onlay impressions	• Fixed partial denture impressions • Crown and bridge impressions • Implant impressions • Inlay and onlay impressions
Preparation	Boil, storage and temper	Powder and water	Two pastes	• Two pastes • Paste and liquid	• Two pastes • Putty	• Two pastes
Mixing surface	No mixing	Flexible mixing bowl	Paper pad	• Paper pad • Automix gun	• Paper pad • Automix gun	• Paper pad • Pentamix™
Spatula	No mixing	Fishtail spatula	Wooden handled, stiff stainless steel spatula	Wooden handled	Stiff stainless steel spatula	Wooden handled
Manipulation	Technique sensitive	Vigorous spatulation	Vigorous spatulation	Vigorous spatulation	Vigorous spatulation	Vigorous spatulation
Placement	In impression tray	Place in tray with spatula	Place in tray with spatula	Place in tray with spatula	Place in tray with spatula	Place in tray with spatula
Patient friendliness	Bulky	Pleasant	Unpleasant	Pleasant	Pleasant	Unpleasant
Ease of removal from patient's mouth	Very easy	Very easy	Easy	Moderate	Moderate	Difficult
Mixing time m – minute(s) s – second(s)	No mixing	Regular set: 1 m Fast: 45 s	45–60 s	45–60 s	45–60 s	30–45 s
Working time m – minute(s) s – second(s)		Regular 3–4.5 m Fast: 1.25–2 m	5–7 m	3 m	2–4 m	2.5 m
Setting time m – minute(s) s – second(s)	5 m	Regular 1–4.5 m Fast: 1–2 m	8–12 m	6–8 m	3–7 m	4.5 m
Shrinkage on setting	High shrinkage	High shrinkage	Moderate to high shrinkage	High to moderate shrinkage	Very low shrinkage	Low shrinkage

FURTHER READING

Dublin Dental Hospital. (2010). *Cross Infection Control Policy*. DDH: Dublin.

Chapter 12

Gypsum materials

DEFINITION

Gypsum (calcium sulphate dihydrate) is a naturally occurring mineral used in dentistry to fabricate models (Figure 12.1a), casts and dies (Figure 12.1b). Calcination is the process of heating the gypsum to dehydrate it (partially or completely) to form calcium sulphate hemihydrate. Plaster and stone are products of the dehydration process. It is the calcination process that determines the strength of the gypsum material. The differences in the types of gypsum are related to the amount of water removed, resulting in varying densities and particle sizes of the material.

Gypsum materials are combined with water and spatulated to create a slurried mixture that is poured into a dental impression (negative reproduction of the teeth and surrounding tissues). It is allowed to set, after which the gypsum and impression are separated, resulting in the positive reproduction of the patient's tooth/teeth, arch and surrounding tissues. Many dental appliances and restorations are constructed extra-orally using models, dies (one tooth) and casts (replicas of the patients tooth/teeth and surrounding tissues).

It is desirable that all gypsum products are strong, compatible with impression materials and waxes and fluid at the time of pouring into the impression; they should also have good dimensional stability.

Powder and water ratios of gypsum products are important. The less water used in the mixture, the stronger the model. Excess water in a mixture of gypsum increases the setting time and reduces the strength and hardness of the final product.

The International Organisation for Standardisation (ISO) has classified gypsum products into the following five types:

Type I	Edentulous impressions and mounting casts on articulators
Type II	Plaster (model)
Type III	Dental stone, die, model
Type IV	Dental stone, die, high strength, low expansion
Type V	Dental stone, high strength, high expansion

Material constituents/composition

- Calcium sulphate dehydrate

GYPSUM MATERIALS

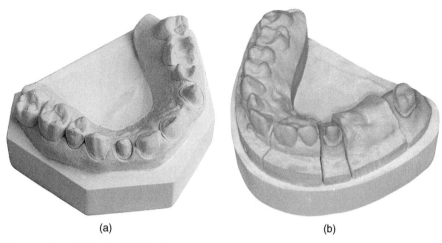

(a)   (b)

Figure 12.1 (a) Model. (b) Model with die.

PLASTER (PLASTER OF PARIS)

Properties

- A calcium sulphate hemihydrate ($CaSO_4, 0.5H_2O$)
- Oldest form of gypsum
- Weakest of all gypsum products
- When mixed with water, it rehardens to a dehydrate

Uses

- Study models
- Casts

Water/powder ratio

- Unspecific

GYPSUM MATERIALS

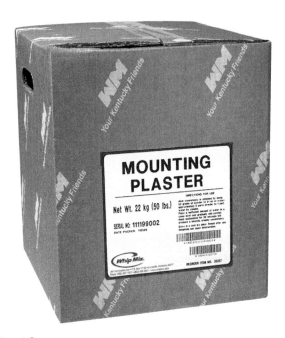

Figure 12.2 Type I Gypsum.

TYPE I – IMPRESSION PLASTER

See Figure 12.2.

Properties

- Good dimensional stability
- Hydrophilic
- Brittle
- High fracture rate

Uses

- Impressions of edentulous patients
- Occlusal registrations

Water/powder ratio

- 60 ml water to 100 grams powder

GYPSUM MATERIALS

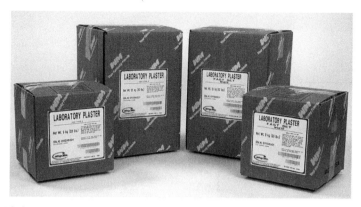

Figure 12.3 Type II Gypsum.

TYPE II – PLASTER (MODEL)

See Figure 12.3.

Properties

- High-grade plaster
- Durable
- Easily manipulated
- Stronger than Type I

Uses

- Study models

Water/powder ratio

- 50 ml water to 100 grams powder

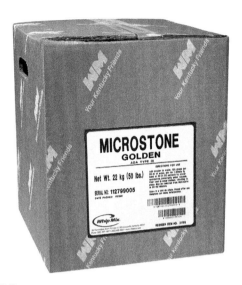

Figure 12.4 Type III Gypsum.

TYPE III – DENTAL STONE, DIE, MODEL

See Figure 12.4.

Properties

- Hard
- Accurate
- Smooth consistency
- Stone is stronger than plaster
- Stone mixture requires less water than plaster due to its small particle size and low porosity
- May appear yellow due to dye material added by the manufacturer

Uses

- Working casts
- Models for partial and complete/full dentures

Water/powder ratio

- 30 ml water to 100 grams powder

TYPE IV – DENTAL STONE, HIGH STRENGTH, HIGH EXPANSION

See Figures 12.5a and 12.5b.

Properties

- Modified alpha-hemihydrate
- Dense
- Stronger than Type III stone
- Stone is stronger than plaster
- Stone mixture requires less water than plaster due to its small particle size and low porosity

Uses

- Wax pattern dies

Water/powder ratio

- 20 ml water to 100 grams powder

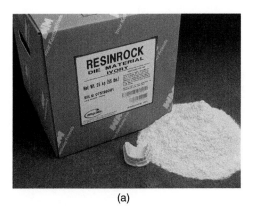
(a)

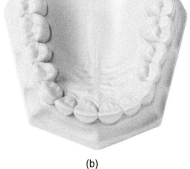
(b)

Figure 12.5 Type IV Gypsum.

TYPE V – DENTAL STONE, DIE, HIGH STRENGTH, LOW EXPANSION

See Figures 12.6a, 12.6b and 12.6c.

Properties

- Newest gypsum added to the American Dental Association (ADA) materials list
- Strongest of the gypsum products
- Stone is stronger than plaster
- Stone mixture requires less water than plaster due to its small particle size and low porosity

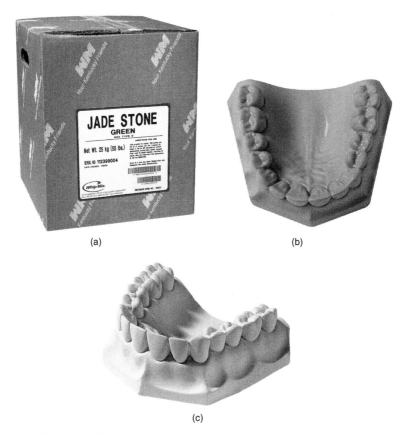

(a)

(b)

(c)

Figure 12.6 Type V Gypsum.

GYPSUM MATERIALS

Uses

- Wax pattern dies for high shrinkage alloys

Water/powder ratio

- 19 ml water to 100 grams powder

Trade names

Type	Trade name	Manufacturer
Type I	Impression Plaster	Whip Mix
Type II	Laboratory Plaster	Whip Mix
Type III	Microstone	Whip Mix
	Quick Stone	Whip Mix
Type IV	Prima Rock	Whip Mix
	Resin Rock	Whip Mix
Type V	Jade Stone	Whip Mix
	Hard Rock	Whip Mix
	Hard Rock	Whip Mix

MANIPULATION (MIXING AND POURING GYPSUM TYPE III INTO AN ALGINATE IMPRESSION)

Wearing personal protective equipment:

Ensure the impression has been properly disinfected prior to the procedure to reduce the risk of cross-infection.

Step 1

- Measure 50 ml of room temperature water in calibrated water measure

Step 2

- Measure 100 grams of plaster into a flexible mixing bowl

Step 3

- Add the gypsum and water together

GYPSUM MATERIALS

Step 4

- Using a flat, wooden-handled, stainless steel spatula, use the tip to initially mix the gypsum and water together (ensure all particles are incorporated into the water)
- Once the materials are incorporated, spatulate in a circular motion rapidly (2 bowl revolutions per second)
- Inadequate mixing of gypsum will affect its final strength
- This initial mix should take no longer than 20 seconds
- Mixing can also be done with a vacuum mixing unit (Figure 12.8d)

Step 5

- Using a laboratory vibrator place the bowl on top to vibrate air bubbles out of the gypsum mixture
- Continue to alternate between mixing and vibrating for the remainder of the mixing time (1 minute)
- Press material against the sides of the bowl during mixing to re-duce/eliminate air bubbles
- Don't over vibrate the material as it can cause additional air bubbles
- Air bubbles present in the final mix will result in voids in the material

Step 6

- The final mix should appear as a thick cream-like consistency

Pouring the model

Step 7

- Pick up a small amount of the gypsum material with the tip of the spatula
- Grasping the handle of the impression tray, gently place the right side of the impression tray on the vibrator

Step 8

- Place a small amount of material in the left side of the impression (in the area of the last tooth in the arch)

GYPSUM MATERIALS

- Allow the vibration from the vibrator to move the gypsum material towards the midline of the arch

Step 9

- Repeat step 8 until the right side is reached

Step 10

- Repeat steps 8 and 9 until the teeth portions of the impression are full

Step 11

- Using the tip of the spatula, add larger increments of gypsum to the impression until the impression tray is full
- Set aside to harden

Creating a base for a cast

Step 12

- Clean the flexible mixing bowl and spatula (*Do not pour excess gypsum down the sink as it may clog the sink – some sinks may have a special trap to catch the gypsum. Excess gypsum may be put in the waste bin*)
- Repeat steps 1 to 6 to create a fresh mix (using less water for the mix (approximately 40 ml) – the base should be thicker so the gypsum material does not 'slump')

Step 13

- If a rubber model former is available, you may fill this with gypsum material
- If a rubber model former is not available, place a glass slab on the work surface and place the gypsum into a patty on the surface

Step 14

- Invert the poured impression onto the rubber model former or the patty of gypsum

GYPSUM MATERIALS

- Pay attention to ensure the impression is parallel to the work surface

Step 15

- Using the tip of the spatula 'pull' up the gypsum material to the level of the alginate of the impression, including in the retromolar and maxillary tuberosity areas

Step 16

- Leave the gypsum material to set – allowing the exothermic reaction to be complete (the material heats up during hardening). The material should feel cold and dry

Step 17

- Separate the gypsum and alginate impression very carefully
- Dispose of the alginate and stock tray in the contaminated waste bin (if using a stainless steel tray, clean and sterilise the tray for re-use)
- (*Do not pour excess gypsum down the sink as it may clog the sink – some sinks may have a special trap to catch the gypsum fitted. Excess gypsum may be put in the waste bin*)

Step 18

- Trim the model using a model trimmer

(Figures 12.7a–q).

Mixing time

- 1 minute

Setting time

The initial set of gypsum is between the commencing of spatulation and when the mixture loses its glossiness (glossiness is lost because the chemical reaction of the hemihydrate uses up the water and the remaining water is pulled into the material). The material is still pliable, but not runny. The initial set takes approximately 8 to 16 minutes.

During the setting of gypsum it returns to its dehydrate state. During this reaction heat is given off (exothermic reaction).

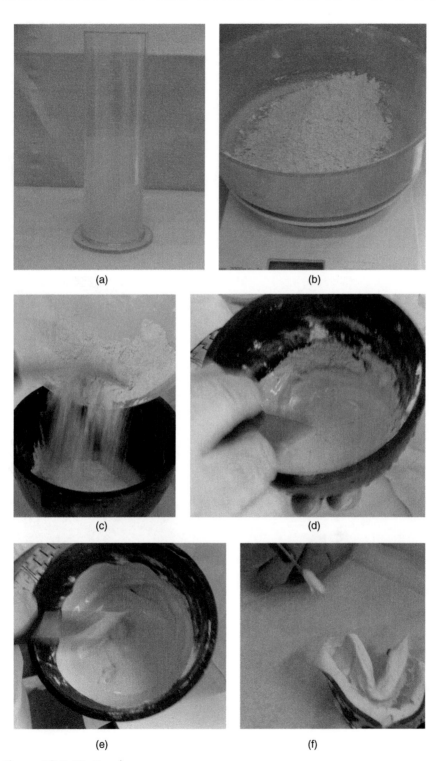

(a)

(b)

(c)

(d)

(e)

(f)

Figure 12.7 (*Continued*)

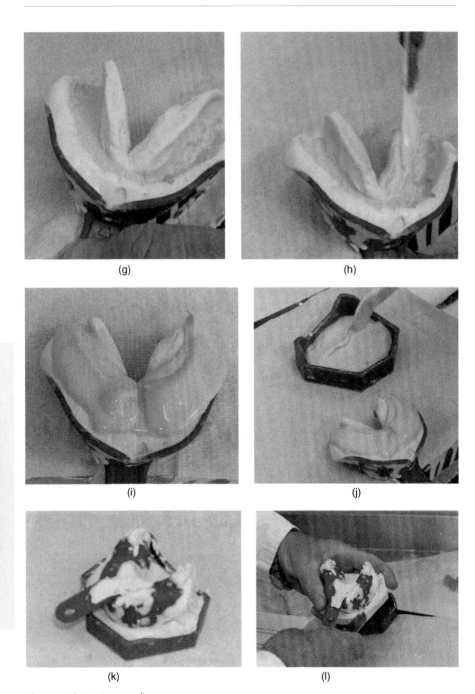

(g)

(h)

(i)

(j)

(k)

(l)

Figure 12.7 (Continued)

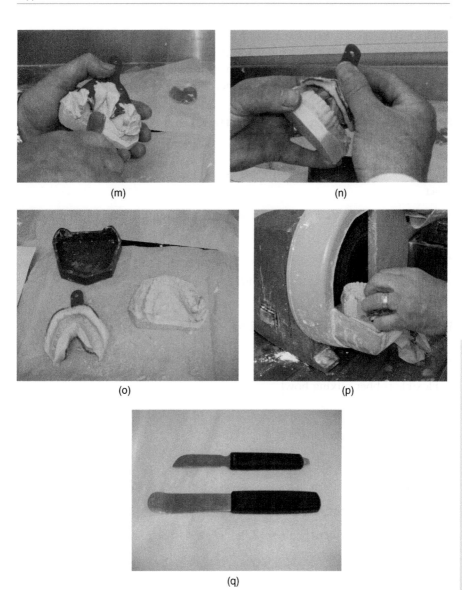

(m)

(n)

(o)

(p)

(q)

Figure 12.7 (a) Step 1 – Water measure (slurry water has been used for photographic purposes). (b) Step 2 – Weigh gypsum material. (c) Step 3 – Add gypsum to water. (d) Step 4 – Commence manipulation. (e) Step 5 – Manipulation to final consistency (using vibrator). (f,g) Step 8 – Loading gypsum into impression using vibrator. (h) Step 9 – Continue adding gypsum until opposite side is reached. (i) Step 11 – Repeat until teeth portions are full 12.7. (j) Step 13 – Fill rubber model former with gypsum. (k) Step 14 – Invert impression onto rubber model former. (l–o) Step 17 – Separate impression and gypsum carefully. (p) Step 18 – Trim model. (q) Plaster spatula and knife.

The final set is reached when all of the heat is gone (the conversion of the hemihydrate to dehydrate is complete). It is important to wait until after the final setting (45–60 minutes) before separating the impression and gypsum. Gypsum gets stronger and harder with increased setting time.

Factors affecting the setting time of gypsum products

- The longer the gypsum and water are spatulated, the faster the material will set
- The higher the temperature and humidity, the shorter the working and setting time
- Powder and water ratio
- Retarders or accelerators added during manufacturing

Instruments and materials used in set-up

- Gypsum material
- Flexible rubber mixing bowl
- Plaster spatula
- Laboratory / plaster knife
- Weighing scale
- Water measure
- Laboratory vibrator (Figures 12.8a and 12.8b)
- Rubber model former (Figures 12.8e), glass slab or paper towel

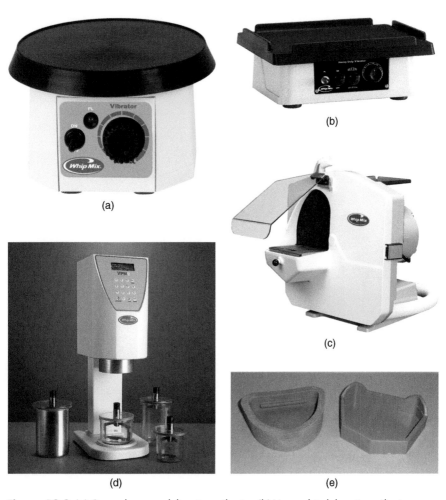

Figure 12.8 (a) General-purpose laboratory vibrator. (b) Heavy-duty laboratory vibrator. (c) Model trimmer. (d) Vacuum mixing unit. (e) Rubber model former.

FURTHER READING

Whipmix. (2009). *Whip Mix Gypsums Physical Properties*. KY: Whipmix. Available at: http://www.whipmix.com/Product_Files/gypum_instructions_1.pdf (Accessed 15 April 2009).

GYPSUM MATERIALS

Chapter 13
Dental waxes

INTRODUCTION

Waxes have a variety of uses within dentistry and are manufactured from various materials, including plants, minerals, animals and synthetic waxes. They can be used both intra- and extra-orally.

Waxes can be divided into three categories: pattern, processing and impression waxes. They are thermoplastic materials that present as solids at room temperature; they can be softened with heat and hardened with cooling.

Waxes are often used in conjunction with dies and models (see Chapter 12) to facilitate construction of various restorations, appliances and prostheses. This chapter does not aim to discuss ways in which wax patterns are created, but instead discusses the various types of waxes and their composition and function (Figure 13.1).

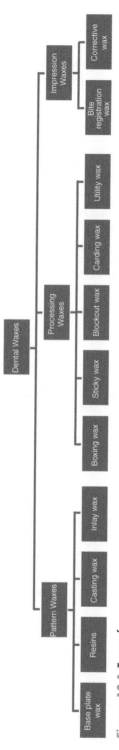

Figure 13.1 Types of waxes.

DENTAL WAXES

PATTERN WAXES

Pattern waxes are used to pattern moulds of various restorations and dental prosthesis. They all burn out without leaving a residue, create smooth surfaces and carve easily.

Wax	Function	Forms available	Constituents
Base plate wax (Figures 13.2a and 13.2b)	• Bite registrations • Hold the position of the teeth in a denture prior to processing • Patterns for orthodontic appliances, occlusal rims and complete/full dentures	• Sheets • Pink or red • Three types of hardness available	• Ceresin • Beeswax • Carauba wax • Synthetic waxes
Resins	• Patterns for restorations	• Chemically cured acrylics • Light-cured composites	• Chemically cured acrylics • Light-cured composites
Casting wax (Figures 13.2c and 13.2d)	• Used for patterns of frameworks for partial dentures	• Sheets, bulk and rods • Blue, pink and white	May contain a combination of: • Paraffin • Cresin • Carnauba • Beeswax
Inlay wax (Figure 13.2e)	• Fabricate patterns of inlays, crowns and pontics	• Cones and sticks • Purple, blue and green • Varying degrees of hardness	May contain a combination of: • Paraffin • Cresin • Carnauba • Beeswax

DENTAL WAXES

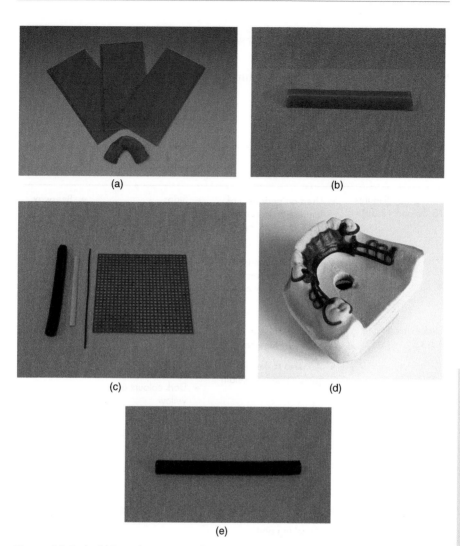

Figure 13.2 (a, b) Baseplate wax. (c, d) Casting wax. (e) Inlay wax.

PROCESSING WAXES

Processing waxes have an auxiliary function in the fabrication of impressions and casts.

DENTAL WAXES

Wax	Function	Forms available	Constituents
Boxing wax (Figures 13.3a and 13.3b)	• Used on periphery of impression to create a 'box' to retain the gypsum • Used on the periphery of an impression tray to reduce irritation to soft tissues	• Strips • Ropes • Green, red and black	• Beeswax • Paraffin • Soft waxes
Sticky wax (Figure 13.3c)	• Temporarily fuse materials together • Adheres to metal, gypsum and porcelain	• Hard rounded sticks • Sheets • Dark colours and yellow	• Beeswax • Rosin
Blockout wax (Figure 13.3d)	• Fill voids and undercuts	• Sheets or disks	• Beeswax • Paraffin • Soft waxes
Carding wax (Figure 13.3e)	• Soldering techniques • Attaching parts	• Sheets and ropes	• Beeswax • Paraffin • Soft waxes
Utility wax (Figures 13.3f and 13.3g)	• Various lab uses • Often used along with boxing wax for similar purposes • Used for orthodontic patients to relieve discomfort from brackets and wires	• Long and short ropes • Red, orange and white	• Beeswax • Paraffin • Soft waxes

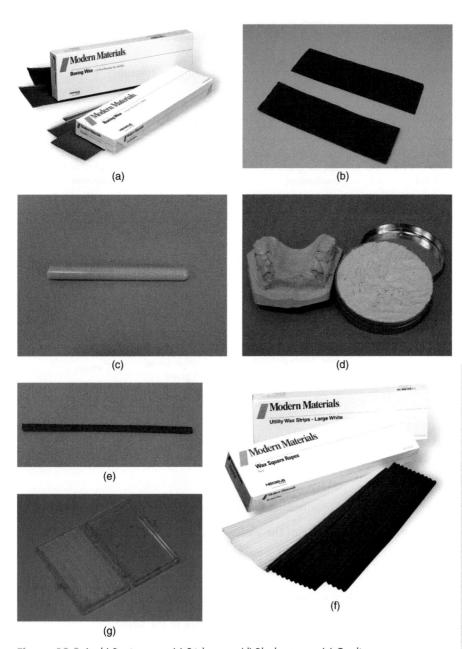

Figure 13.3 (a, b) Boxing wax. (c) Sticky wax. (d) Blockout wax. (e) Carding wax. (f, g) Utility wax.

Impression waxes are used intra-orally for taking impressions.

Wax	Function	Forms available	Constituents
Bite registration wax (Figure 13.4a)	• Bite registrations of opposing arches (replication)	• Sheets • Sticks • Orange, white and green	May contain a combination of: • Beeswax • Paraffin • Ceresin • Oils • Aluminium particles • Copper particles
Corrective wax (Figure 13.4b)	• Used over an original impression to record soft tissue details in edentulous patients	• Sheets • Sticks • Orange, white and green	May contain a combination of: • Paraffin • Ceresin • Metallic particles • Castor oil

Methods for softening wax prior to use include the following:

Water bath (Figure 13.5a)

- Regular and uniform softening by maintaining constant temperature
- Waxes may absorb some of the water affecting their properties

Bunsen burner (Figure 13.5b)

- Care must be taken to soften the wax evenly and not melt it
- Hold the wax in the area above the flame, not in the flame

Wax annealer (Figure 13.5c)

- Specialised oven used to soften the wax
- Keeps the wax at a constant temperature

DENTAL WAXES

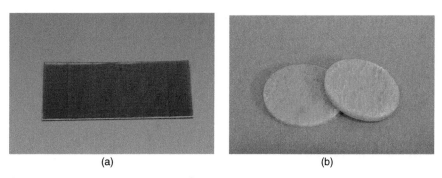

Figure 13.4 (a) Bite registration wax. (b) Corrective wax.

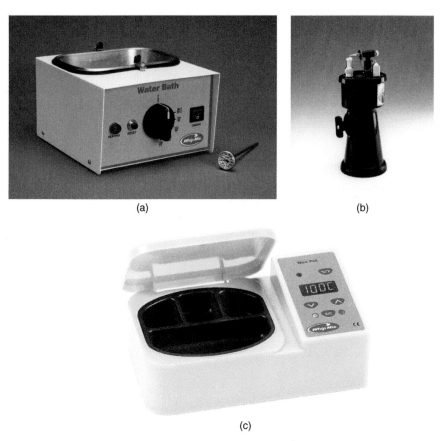

Figure 13.5 (a) Water bath. (b) Bunsen burner. (c) Wax annealer.

Instruments and materials used in set-up

- Choice of wax
- Choice of heat source
- Wax knife
- Le Cron carver
- Flat plastic instrument
- Bowl of cool water

DENTAL WAXES

Chapter 14
Material safety data sheets

Dental materials contain various chemicals that are potentially hazardous. Manufacturers of chemicals are required legally to provide a Material Safety Data Sheet (MSDS) for each material that contains a hazardous chemical, as well as label the product. MSDSs outline potential hazards involved when working with these materials. Manufacturers have evaluated the potential risks of the material and use the MSDS to convey this information.

It is the responsibility of the dental team, often the responsibility of the dental nurse, to maintain a comprehensive file of the MSDSs for every material used within the surgery. The file must be easily accessed by the whole dental team and complete with all MSDSs. These files are available from the manufacturer and often exist on the internet.

Labelling hazardous containers and staff training are the key to working safely around hazardous chemicals. Employees must have the education to understand the potential risks involved when working with chemicals, safe handling and what action to take in the event of an emergency. Every time there is a new material introduced into the dental surgery, all staff must be made aware of the composition and possible hazards. Appropriate training should be provided for its use if required.

The MSDS is primarily designed to be of use to those who work with a substance or treat those who have been injured by accidental exposure or misuse of a product.

DENTAL STAFF TRAINING

Training for staff should involve the understanding of:

- Where the MSDS file is kept
- Which staff member is in charge of keeping it up-to-date and informing other staff of changes
- How to read and understand an MSDS
- Understand and identify hazardous signs
- What actions to take in the event of an emergency involving a hazardous chemical
- The importance of Personal Protective Equipment (PPE)
- Safe handling of chemicals

INFORMATION CONTAINED IN MSDS

MSDS will contain variations of the following information:

- Name and address of the manufacturer
- Identification of the material (trade name and chemical name)
- Physical and chemical composition (e.g. boiling point, vapour pressure, appearance)
- Hazardous ingredients
- Toxicological information
- Health hazard data (signs and symptoms of exposure and routes of entry)
- Emergency first aid measures
- Fire and explosion information (Flash point and flammable limits)
- Reactivity data (e.g. stability, incompatibility, decomposition by-products)
- Safe disposal information
- Spillage clean up and information
- Safe handling and safe storage information
- Transportation considerations
- Preparation date of MSDS

The dental team should also maintain a log outlining the name of each item containing hazardous chemical and where they are stored.

Appendices 14.1 and 14.2 are examples of typical MSDSs.

MATERIAL SAFETY DATA SHEETS

Appendix 14.1

MATERIAL SAFETY DATA SHEET [according to GHS & NOHSC: 2011(2003)]   **Page 1 of 5**
Product: PERMITE C CAPSULES; LOJIC + CAPSULES; GS-80 CAPSULES;
GS-80 SPHERICAL CAPSULES; F400 CAPSULES; ULTRACAPS +
AND ULTRACAPS S
Date / Revised: 31.01.2006   Revision: 4

1. Substance / Preparation and Company name

Product Name: Permite C Capsules; Lojic + Capsules; GS-80 Capsules, GS-80 Spherical
                     Capsules; F400 Capsules; Ultracaps + and Ultracaps S

Recommended use: For filling of cavitated teeth by dental professionals.

Manufacturer / Supplier

SDI Limited   SDI Inc.
5-9 Brunsdon Street, Bayswater   729 N.Route 83, Suite 315
Victoria, 3153, Australia   Bensenville 60106 IL, USA

Telephone: **Telephone:**

+61 3 8727 7111 (Business hours)   630 238 8300 (Business hours)

Southern Dental Industries Ltd   SDI Brasil Indústria e Comércio Ltda
Block 8, St Johns Court   Rua Dr. Virgílio de Carvalho Pinto, 612
Swords Road   Pinheiros, São Paulo, 05415-020
Santry, Dublin 9, Ireland   Brasil

Telephone: **Telephone:**

+353 1 886 9577 (Business Hours)   +(5511) 3031 1700 (Business Hours)

Emergency contact number: +61 3 8727 7111

2. Composition / Information on ingredients

Hazardous ingredient:	Wt.%	CAS No.	EEC No.	Index No.
Compartment 1:				
Mercury, metallic	100	7439-97-6	231-106-7	080-001-00
(40-50% of total product)				
Compartment 2:				
Non toxic alloy powder	100			

3. Hazard Identification:

These products contain mercury. It is toxic if inhaled and acute exposure may cause allergic reactions
including dermatitis, digestion and respiratory disorders.

California Prop 65 Warning   This product contains mercury, a chemical known to the State of
                                     California to cause birth defects or other reproductive harm.

	T	Toxic
Risk phrases:	**23**	Toxic by inhalation
	33	Danger of cumulative effects
Safety phrases:	**1/2**	Keep locked up and out of reach of children
	7	Keep container tightly closed.
	9	Keep container in a well ventilated place.
	45	In case of accident or if you feel unwell, contact a doctor or Poisons Information Centre immediately (show the label where possible).

MATERIAL SAFETY DATA SHEET [according to GHS & NOHSC: 2011(2003)]   **Page 2 of 5**
Product: PERMITE C CAPSULES; LOJIC + CAPSULES; GS-80 CAPSULES;
**   GS-80 SPHERICAL CAPSULES; F400 CAPSULES; ULTRACAPS +**
**   AND ULTRACAPS S**
Date / Revised: 31.01.2006   **Revision: 4**

---

4.   First Aid Measures

General advice: Contains metallic mercury. In case of accident or if you feel unwell, seek medical advice immediately (show label where possible).

If inhaled: Toxic by inhalation.   Remove to fresh air.   Seek medical attention.   If not breathing give artificial respiration.

                       May cause respiratory disorders including inflammation and fluid retention. Inhalation of mercury vapours at high concentration can cause dyspnea, coughing, fever, severe nausea, vomiting, excess salivation, kidney damage with renal shutdown.

If ingested: Call a physician immediately.   Give large amounts of water.

On skin contact: Wash skin with soap and water.   Remove contaminated clothing.   May cause irritation and allergic reaction.

On contact with eyes: Wash with clear, tepid water. If irritation persists, obtain medical attention. May cause irritation and allergic reaction.

---

5.   Fire Fighting Measures

Suitable extinguishing media: As for adjacent fire.   Avoid direct water stream.   Do not allow water runoff to enter sewers and waterways.   Remove product from the fire area if this can be done without risk.

Special protective equipment: In fires involving large quantities of product, use self-contained breathing apparatus and full protective clothing.

Further information: Hazardous decomposition products may be produced.   (Sec. 10).

---

6.   Accidental Release Measures

Spillages: Mercury presents a health hazard if incorrectly handled. Spillages of mercury should be removed immediately, including from places which are difficult to access. Use a plastic syringe to draw it up. Smaller quantities can be covered by sulphur powder and removed. Avoid inhalation of the vapour.

Personal precautions: Wear appropriate MSHA approved respirator, gloves, safety goggles and protective clothing to prevent skin contact.

Environmental precautions: Prevent any spillage from entering drains or waterways.

Methods for cleaning up: Avoid contact with skin and eyes. Pick up with dust pan or method that does not break up mercury into smaller droplets, etc. Store in a sealed plastic container, away from heat and flame, until disposal via an approved Recycler.

MATERIAL SAFETY DATA SHEETS

7. Handling and storage

Handling
Do not breathe powder and avoid exposed mercury surfaces.   Wear appropriate gloves, goggles, and protective clothing to prevent skin contact.   Wash thoroughly after handling.   Keep away from food, drink and around animal feed stuffs.

Storage
Keep container tightly closed and dry.   Storage in large quantities (as in warehouse) should be in a ventilated, cool area.   Do not store in metal containers.   Keep away from sources of ignition and elevated temperatures, recommended <25°C.

8. Exposure controls and personal protection

8-Hour TWAs: Mercury - 0.025 mg/m^3 (Skin) (ACGIH);   0.05 mg/m^3 (Skin) (OSHA/UK & NOHSC/Australia); 0.1 mg/m^3 (Short term) (Germany);
Silver -   0.01 mg/m^3 (OSHA/Germany); 0.1 mg/m^3 (ACGIH/U.K. & NOHSC/Australia)
Tin -   2 mg/m^3 (OSHA/ACGIH/Germany & NOHSC/Australia); 5 mg/m^3 (U.K.);
Copper - 1 mg/m^3 (OSHA/ACGIH/Germany/UK & NOHSC/Australia)
Indium - 0.1 mg/m^3 (OSHA/UK & NOHSC/Australia)
Zinc -   1 mg/m^3 (ACGIH)

These levels are not anticipated under foreseeable use conditions.

Personal protective equipment

Respiratory equipment: None required under normal use conditions.

Hand protection: Impervious gloves.

Eye protection: Safety goggles.

General safety and hygiene measures: Use only as directed. Wash hands after use.

9. Physical and chemical properties

Form and Colour: Silver alloy powder and mercury in separate compartments of a plastic capsule.

Odour:	Odourless
Melting point / melting range:	(Mercury): -38.9°C
Boiling point / boiling range:	(Mercury): 356.6°C
Flash point:	Not applicable
Explosion limits:	Not applicable
Ignition temperature:	Not applicable
Vapour pressure:	(Mercury) 0.0012 mmHg at 20°C
Specific Gravity:	(Mercury) 13.6 g/cm^3
% Volatiles:	Not applicable
Solubility in water:	Insoluble
Solubility in other solvents:	Insoluble in alcohol
pH value:	Not available
Octanol / water partition coefficient (log POW):	Not determined
Viscosity:	Not determined
Other information:	N/A

MATERIAL SAFETY DATA SHEETS

10. Stability and Reactivity

Thermal decomposition: No decomposition under normal conditions

Substance(s) to avoid: Strong oxidizers

Hazardous reactions: Mixtures of mercury with acetylene, ammonia, chlorine dioxide, methyl azide, chlorates, nitrates, or hot sulfuric acid can be explosive. Readily amalgamates with most metals.

Hazardous decomposition products: Slightly volatile at room temperature, atmospheric pressure. When exposed to high temperatures, mercury vaporizes to extremely toxic fumes.

11. Toxicological information

Critical hazards to man: Toxic by inhalation.   Acute exposure may cause allergic reactions including dermatitis, digestion and respiratory disorders.

Critical hazards to the environment: Not available.

None available regarding product.   Some information supplied for ingredient(s).

LCLo / Inhalation / Rabbit: (Mercury) 29 mg/m^3/30 Hour

Chronic Health Effects: Inhalation of mercury vapours, dusts or organic vapours, or skin absorption or mercury over long periods can cause mercurialism.   Symptoms include tremors, inflammation of mouth and gums, excessive salivation, stomatitis, blue lines on gums, pain and numbness in extremities, weight loss, mental depression, and nervousness.   Exposure may aggravate kidney disorders, chronic respiratory disease and nervous system disorders.

12. Ecological information

German "Wassergefaehrdungs Klasse (WGK):3
This product must not enter effluent, ground water, surface water or the soil.

13. Disposal considerations

Product: Dispose of in accordance with local regulations.

***The 1991 Environmental Protection* (Duty of Care) *Regulations SI No. 2839 and amendments should be noted* (United Kingdom).**

14. Transport information

This product is not considered to be a dangerous good within the meaning of transportation regulations.
Labelled according to ISO 24234:2004(E) – Mercury and alloys for dental amalgam.

15. Regulatory information

These products are regulated by:

TGA
Medical Devices Directives 93/42/EEC
FDA
National regulations

16. Other information

Preparation of MSDS:

Prepared by: SDI Limited   **Phone Number:**
5-9 Brunsdon Street, Bayswater   +61 3 8727 7111
Victoria, 3153, Australia

The information contained in the Material Safety Data Sheet is based on data considered to be accurate, however, no warranty is expressed or implied regarding the accuracy of the data or the results to be obtained from the use thereof.

Department issuing MSDS: Research and Development
Contact: Operations Director

Appendix 14.2

 MATERIAL SAFETY DATA SHEET   [according to GHS & NOHSC:2011(2003)]   **Page 1 of 4**
Product: GLACIER; WAVE, WAVE MV, WAVE HV, ROK, ICE AND LC OPAQUER
Date / Revised: 01.06.2006   **Revision: 5**

---

1. **Substance / Preparation and Company name**

    Product Name: Glacier; Wave; Wave MV; Wave HV; ROK, ICE and LC Opaquer

    Recommended use: For filling of cavita ted teeth by dental professionals.

    Manufacturer / Supplier

    S DI Limited   S DI Inc.
    5-9 Brunsdon Street, Bayswater   729 N.Route 83, Suite 315
    Victoria, 3153, Australia   Bensenville 60106 IL, USA

    Telephone: **Telephone:**

    +61 3 8727 7111 (Business hours)   630 238 8300 (Business hours)

    Southern Dental Industries Ltd   SDI Brasil Indústria e Comércio Ltda
    Block 8, St Johns Court   Rua Dr. Virgílio de Carvalho Pinto, 612
    S words R oad   P inheiros, São Paulo, 05415-020
    Santry, Dublin 9, Ireland   Brasil

    Telephone: **Telephone:**

    +353 1 886 9577 (Business Hours)   +(5511) 3031 1700 (Business Hours)

    Emergency contact number: +61 3 8727 7111

---

2. **Composition / Information on ingredients**

Composition:	CAS No.	Wt. %
Acrylic monomer	-	18.0 – 40.0
Balance ingredient (non-hazardous)		60.0 – 82.0

---

3. **Hazard Identification**

    Products may cause irritation to the skin, eye and mucous membrane. Ingestion of unpolymerised material may cause gastric irritation. In isolated cases, contact allergies have been reported with acrylic resins. Anyone with known history of resin allergies are advised to seek the advice of a specialist before use.

    Risk phrases - **36/37/38**:   Irritating to eyes, respiratory system and skin.

    Safety phrases - **26/28**:   In case of contact with eyes, rinse immediately with plenty of water and seek medical advice. After contact with skin, wash immediately with soap and water.

    - **3/15/16**:   Keep in a cool place, away from heat and sources of ignition.

    - **2**:   Keep out of reach of children.

SDI ***MATERIAL SAFETY DATA SHEET*** [according to GHS & NOHSC:2011(2003)] **Page 2 of 4**
Product: GLACIER; WAVE, WAVE MV, WAVE HV, ROK, ICE AND LC OPAQUER
Date / Revised: 01.06.2006   **Revision: 5**

4. First Aid Measures

Eye (contact):   Flush opened eye with running water for at least 5 minutes.   Seek medical
                          attention.

Skin (contact):   Remove contaminated clothing.   Wash skin with soap and water.   In case of
                          allergic reaction, seek medical attention.

Ingestion: Seek medical attention.

Inhalation: None expected.

5. Fire Fighting Measures

Suitable extinguishing media: Sand, chemical foam, carbon dioxide, dry chemicals.

Unusual Fire and Explosion
              Hazards: Heat can cause polymerization with rapid release of energy which may
                          melt the container.

Special protective equipment: No special measures required for small quantity (less than 1 kg).   For
                          large quantity, wear approved respirat or and protective gear. Use
                          water spray to cool container.

6. Accidental Release Measures

Personal precautions: Not required.

Environmental precautions: Prevent any spillage from entering waterways, drains or sewage
                            system.

Methods for cleaning up: Scoop up bulk material and transfer to containers for disposal.

7. Handling and storage

Handling
Replace caps immediately after use.

Storage
Store in a cool place at temperatures between 10°C and 25°C (50° - 77°F).   Keep out of direct light.

8. Exposure controls and personal protection

Respiratory protection: None required under normal conditions of use

Hand protection: Rubber, latex or PVC gloves.

Eye protection: Not absolutely necessary

General safety and hygiene measures: Follow good housekeeping practices and good industrial
                                     hygiene in handling this material.   Remove any naked lights
                                     or strong heat sources.

MATERIAL SAFETY DATA SHEETS

9.   Physical and chemical properties

Appearance:	Tooth coloured viscous / flowable paste.
Odour:	Ester like.
Boiling point:	Gel before boiling.
Melting point:	Not established.
Specific gravity:	1.5 - 2.0
Flash point:	Not established.
Flammable:	Not established.
Autoflammability:	Do not self ignite.
Explosive properties:	Do not present an explosion hazard.
Oxidizing properties:	Not established.
Vapour pressure (@ 20 °C):	0 mbar
Relative density:	Not established.
Solubility:	Insoluble in water.

10. Stability and Reactivity

Stability:	Stable under normal conditions.
Conditions to avoid:	Avoid heat, ignition sources, aging, contamination and intense visible light.
Materials to avoid:	Free radical formers, e.g. peroxides, reducing substances and / or heavy metals ions.
Hazardous decomposition products:	None under normal conditions. Oxides of carbon when burned.
Hazardous reactivity (polymerization):	Heat and intense light can cause polymerization. Spontaneous polymerization may occur in the presence of radical formers. May polymerize under these conditions with heat evolution.

11. Toxicological information

Acute toxicity:	May be irritating to skin, eye and mucous membrane.
Sensitization:	No sensitizing effect known. In isolated cases contact allergies have been reported.
Inhalation:	None expected.

12. Ecological information

Self assessment:	Slightly hazardous for water. Do not allow large quantities to reach sewage system and waterways.

MATERIAL SAFETY DATA SHEETS

SDI

MATERIAL SAFETY DATA SHEET   [according to GHS & NOHSC:2011(2003)]   **Page 4 of 4**
Product: GLACIER; WAVE, WAVE MV, WAVE HV, ROK, ICE AND LC OPAQUER
Date / Revised: 01.06.2006   **Revision: 5**

13. Disposal considerations

Dispose of in accordance with local official regulations.

14. Transport information

Glacier, Wave, Wave MV, Wave   HV, Rok, Ice and LC Opaquer are not classified as Dangerous Goods for air, sea, rail or road transport.

15. Regulatory information

These products are regulated by:

TGA
Medical Devices 93/42/EEC
FDA
National regulations

16. Other information

The information provided herein is given in good faith, but no warranty expressed or implied is made.

Prepared by: SDI Limited   **Phone Number:**
                  5-9 Brunsdon Street, Bayswater   +61 3 8727 7111
                  Victoria, 3153, Australia

Department issuing MSDS: Research and Development
Contact: Operations Director

MATERIAL SAFETY DATA SHEETS

Chapter 15

Introduction to four-handed dentistry

> *Work smarter not harder*

Four-handed dentistry combined with good ergonomics is a team concept practiced to increase efficiency of dental treatment, reduce stress and fatigue and increase patient comfort. It is based on the idea that using chairside time more efficiently will not only create more time, but also foster a team approach to providing patient care.

The following are central to the concept of four-handed dentistry:

- Position of the operator, dental nurse and patient

- Individual skills

- Organisation

- Equipment ergonomics and arrangement

This chapter will introduce the concept of four-handed dentistry in relation to the transfer of dental materials. It does not aim to be an exhaustive resource for the dental professional.

OPERATOR, DENTAL NURSE, PATIENT AND EQUIPMENT POSITIONING

The positioning of the operator, dental nurse and patient is determined by the procedure and which quadrant it is located in. All individuals should be seated throughout all dental procedures.

Operator (Figure 15.1)
The operator should be positioned with:

- Thighs parallel to the floor
- Feet flat on the floor
- Neck and back straight
- Forearms parallel to the floor

The operator's stool should:

- Be mobile

INTRODUCTION TO FOUR-HANDED DENTISTRY

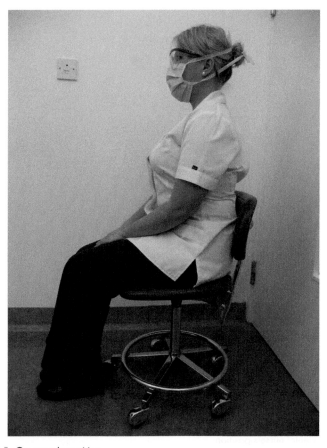

Figure 15.1 Operator's position.

- Have a stable base
- Have a height adjustment lever
- Have back support that can be vertically and horizontally adjusted
- Be padded to reduce the pressure on the thighs and back
- Be covered with a material that allows disinfection without ruining the material

Dental nurse (Figure 15.2)

The dental nurse should be positioned with:

- Thighs parallel to the floor
- Neck and back straight

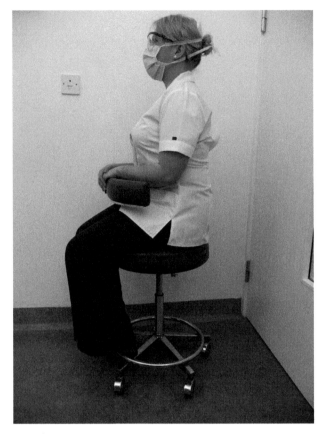

Figure 15.2 Dental nurse's position.

- Forearms parallel to the floor
- Feet rested on the ring of the stool (this is because the dental nurse should be seated 4–6 inches higher than the operator)
- Feet directed towards the top of the patient's chair and body close to the patient's chair
- Body positioned so that the dental nurse can reach the treatment area, static area and transfer zone as well as positioned to allow observation of the patient

The dental nurse's stool should:

- Be mobile with a stable base
- Have a padded seat to reduce pressure on thighs and back
- Have a ring at the bottom to support the dental nurse's feet

- Have a lever to adjust the height

- Have a padded arm to provide body support during movements and while stationary. The padded arm should be positioned just under the dental nurse's rib cage and should not be used as an armrest

- Be covered with a material that allows disinfection without ruining the material

Patient's positioning

The patient should be positioned:

- In the supine position

- With their head at the very top of the headrest

- With their head slightly tilted to the left or right, depending on which quadrant treatment is taking place

- When working in the mandibular arch, the chair must be slightly lowered and the chair back slightly elevated (the operator's arms should still be parallel to the floor)

The patient's chair should:

- Have a thin back to facilitate the operator's legs under the chair and forearms to be parallel to the floor

- Have a rigid solid frame, supporting the patient's back

- Be covered with a material that allows disinfection without ruining the material

- Have adjustment buttons accessible for both the operator and dental nurse (by fingertips and feet)

- Have a base that allows rotation

> Improper seating positions may cause damage to circulation in lower limbs and cause fatigue, stress and lower back pain

The dental unit should be:

- Positioned so it does not interfere with the operator and dental nurse's zones

- Accessible to both the operator and the dental nurse

- Positioned over the patient trans-thoracically

INTRODUCTION TO FOUR-HANDED DENTISTRY

MOVEMENTS

One of the aims of four-handed dentistry is to reduce the amount of unnecessary movements in order to reduce fatigue and stress on the operator and dental nurse. The face of a clock is used to describe the movements of the operator and dental nurse while practising four-handed dentistry.

Both the operator and the dental nurse must be aware of the visibility requirements of each other and do their best to maintain a working field where both can see.

The following describes the movement zones for a *right-handed* operator and a right-handed dental nurse during treatment utilising four-handed dentistry (Figure 15.3):

7:00–12:00	Operator's zone
12:00–2:00	Static zone (this is where mobile cabinets, nitrous oxide machines, blood pressure equipment, etc. should be placed)
2:00–4:00	Dental nurse's zone
4:00–7:00	Transfer zone (this is where the dental unit is positioned and the area for instrument and material transfer)

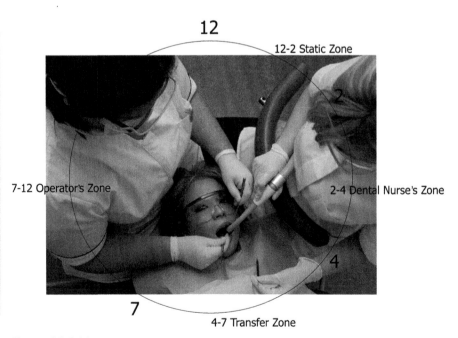

Figure 15.3 Movement zones.

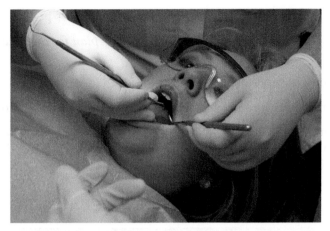

Figure 15.4 Operator maintaining a fulcrum while rotating wrist.

During the transfer of instruments and materials, it is the dental nurse that should be doing the majority of the movements, the operator stays mostly in a static position and the dental nurse facilitates their needs. The main movement of the operator is movement of their wrists and fingers (Figure 15.4). The dental nurse should be aware of the whole picture – the operatory/surgery, instruments, materials, positions, light and patient. This allows the dentist to concentrate on the patient and the oral cavity.

The effective use of the dental nurse depends on the dentist's training on how to utilise a dental nurse's skills and the individual training of the dental nurse.

During treatment, the dental nurse should not leave the patient's side. It is their responsibility for the organisation and preparation of the operatory/surgery. If the operatory/surgery is not properly prepared and the dental nurse is running to fetch forgotten items, this reduces the efficiency of treatment and the standard of care that the patient receives.

Efficient four-handed dentistry is also dependent upon operatory/surgery design, equipment, staff resources, appointment scheduling and inventory systems. If there is a deficiency in any of the above, this will reduce the efficiency of four-handed dentistry.

The following are points that will aid in facilitating the smooth execution of four-handed dentistry:

- Both the operator and the dental nurse must be seated throughout treatment
- Remove any unnecessary items from the operatory/surgery as they impede efficiency by cluttering working areas
- Rinse the patient's mouth with the air-water syringe and high-volume suction

- Have colour-coded trays for each procedure that are set up prior to treatment

- Have tray set-ups standardised and minimalist – *plan for the usual not the unusual*

- Keep multiple operatories/surgeries standardised in organisation

- If equipment is used routinely, there should be one in each operatory

- If equipment, instruments or materials are used occasionally, store them in a mobile trolley that allows them to be easily transferred between operatories/surgeries

PASSING AND RECEIVING INSTRUMENTS AND MATERIALS

The efficient passing and receiving of instruments and materials between the operator and the dental nurse requires exceptional teamwork. The dental nurse must anticipate the operator's needs without delay. After working as a team for a period of time, the dental nurse should become familiar with the sequence of instruments and materials routinely used by the operator and have a complete set-up organised prior to seating the patient.

Instruments and materials are transferred in the transfer zone, near the chin of the patient (instruments should not be passed or exchanged over the patients face for safety reasons). The operator maintains the ready position, and the dental nurse places and retrieves instruments and materials from their hands. The operator pivots the fulcrum and wrist from the working position to the transfer position. The dental nurse's movements involve the wrist, fingers and elbow.

Organisation of instruments and materials by the dental nurse is imperative to facilitate the smooth transfer between the dental nurse and the operator. Armamentarium should be organised left to right in the order of use and re-turned to their original spots after use for ease of retrieval. When assisting a right-handed operator, the dental nurse transfers with the left arm and aspirates/suctions with the right arm (Figures 15.5a and 15.5b).

When exchanging instruments or materials, the dental nurse picks up the item to be transferred with the left hand. The following describes the transfer of a hand instrument between the operator and the dental nurse:

- The dental nurse grasps the hand instrument by the non-working end (grasped between the thumb and first forefinger; Figure 15.6)

- The instrument is extended to the operator parallel to the instrument that the operator is using (Figure 15.7)

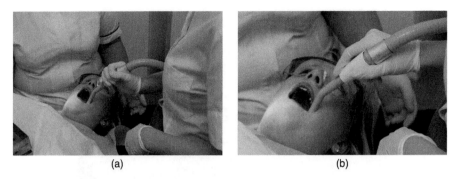

(a)   (b)

Figure 15.5 (a) Palm grasp of the high-volume suction. (b) Pen grasp of the high-volume suction.

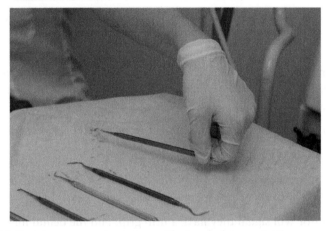

Figure 15.6 Dental nurse preparing instrument for transfer by grasping the non-working end.

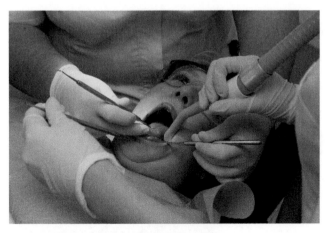

Figure 15.7 Instrument extended to the operator (parallel).

INTRODUCTION TO FOUR-HANDED DENTISTRY

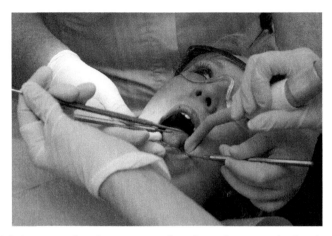

Figure 15.8 Operator rolling their wrist away from the working area, the dental nurse receiving instrument with the little finger and transferring new instrument.

- The operator rolls wrist slightly away from the working area (maintaining fulcrum). This is the signal to the dental nurse that they are ready to transfer instruments

- The dental nurse extends the little finger to receive the instrument

- The dental nurse grasps the used instrument with the little finger

- The new instrument is placed into the operator's hand (as the dental nurse retrieves the instrument by the non-working end; Figure 15.8)

- The operator will signal they have a firm grip, and the dental nurse releases the instrument (Figure 15.9)

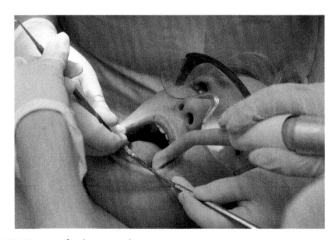

Figure 15.9 Operator firmly grasps the instrument.

INTRODUCTION TO FOUR-HANDED DENTISTRY

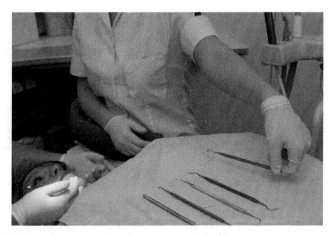

Figure 15.10 Dental nurse returning instrument to original location.

* The dental nurse returns the used instrument to its original location on the tray and lifts the next one by the non-working end, preparing to repeat the above sequence (Figure 15.10)

If transferring instruments such as extraction forceps, the handle should be extended to the operator first (Figure 15.11a and 15.11b).

Dental materials are also transferred in the transfer zone. Understanding and anticipating the sequence of events during a procedure will assist in prompting the execution of the mix. The mixing surface (i.e. waxed paper pad, glass slab or dappen dish) is extended to the operator along with the appropriate applicator (Figure 15.12a). The 3-in-1/air-water syringe is held in the other hand to assist in drying the area prior to placement. Once the area is dried, a piece of gauze should be held to wipe excess material from the operator's *blunt* instrument (this should not be done if the instrument is sharp; Figure 15.12b).

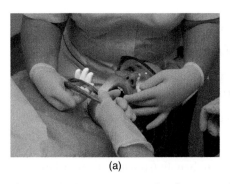
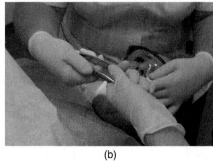

(a)   (b)

Figure 15.11 Instrument transfer of extraction forceps.

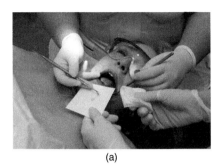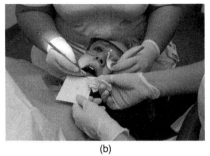

(a)   (b)

Figure 15.12 (a) Transfer of dental material. (b) Wiping excess material from **blunt** instrument.

The following are steps to take to achieve efficient, four-handed dentistry:

- Excellent advance treatment planning and clear recording in the patient's chart enables the dental nurse to be prepared
- The equipment within the dental surgery must be designed in an ergonomically friendly fashion to reduce unnecessary motions
- The dental team and patient must be seated in ergonomically desirable positions
- Utilise preset treatment trays and well-organised surgeries/operatories

The operator must:

- Communicate verbally and non-verbally
- Avoid twisting and turning instruments during transfers
- Avoid 'grabbing' instruments during transfers

The dental nurse must:

- Understand and prepare for the sequence of treatment
- Recognise and anticipate the needs of the operator and the patient
- Anticipate when the usual becomes the unusual and change sequences and prepare alternative materials and instruments
- Keep working areas tidy and organised

With good communication, teamwork and practice, the dental team can execute the principles of four-handed dentistry to benefit from less stress fatigue, increase their efficiency and make the treatment more comfortable for the patient.

Index

Printed and bound by CPI Group (UK) Ltd, Croydon, CR0 4YY